Anti-Inflammatory Diet For Women Over 60

A Complete Guide for Senior Women to Reduce Inflammation, Boost Energy, and Age Gracefully

By

Olivia Stokes

Dear Reader,

Welcome to ***ANTI-INFLAMMATORY DIET FOR WOMEN OVER 60***.

I'm Olivia Stokes, a nutritionist deeply committed to helping women thrive through the transformative power of healthy eating. With years of experience and a passion for promoting vibrant living, I've designed this guide to address the unique nutritional needs of women over 60.

Understanding the vital role that personalized nutrition plays in supporting overall health, I am excited to share a selection of nourishing and flavorful recipes tailored to reduce inflammation and enhance well-being. Each recipe in this book has been thoughtfully chosen to align with anti-inflammatory principles, while also addressing common health concerns that may arise later in life.

I've poured my heart and expertise into this book, and I truly hope it inspires you to take charge of your health and enjoy the benefits of a balanced, anti-inflammatory lifestyle. As you explore these pages, I invite you to embrace this journey with me, discovering new ways to nourish your body and spirit.

Your feedback is incredibly important to me. It helps me grow as an author and guides others on their path to better health. I warmly encourage you to share your thoughts and experiences by leaving a review on Amazon. Your words will not only support my efforts but also help others make informed decisions about their wellness journey.

Thank you for choosing this book. Together, let's embark on a path toward a healthier, happier you.

Warm regards,

Olivia Stokes

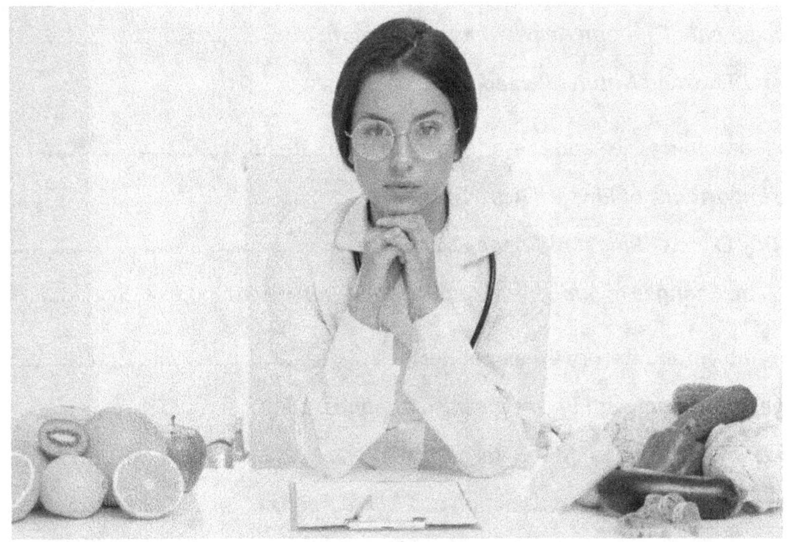

Table of Contents

Introduction

An injury, an illness, or a stimulus that is damaging to the body might cause the body to respond naturally by inflaming itself. It is a component of the defense mechanism maintained by the immune system, which works to protect and cure the body. However, as we age, inflammation can become chronic, leading to a variety of health issues that affect overall well-being. This type of long-term, low-grade inflammation is often referred to as "inflammaging" and is closely linked to the aging process. The aging body undergoes numerous changes at the cellular level, which make it more susceptible to inflammation. Hormonal shifts, particularly the decline in estrogen after menopause, play a significant role in this process. Estrogen has anti-inflammatory properties, and its decrease can trigger a rise in inflammation, affecting various systems in the body. Additionally, the immune system weakens with age, leading to what is known as "immunosenescence." This results in a reduced ability to combat infections and heal injuries effectively, while simultaneously increasing the likelihood of chronic inflammation. Inflammation doesn't just impact the immune system; it has a profound effect on many of the body's vital functions. In women over 60, this can manifest as joint pain, fatigue, and a heightened danger of chronic conditions like cardiovascular disease, diabetes, and neurodegenerative disorders like Alzheimer's. The accumulation of years of oxidative stress, poor dietary habits, and a sedentary lifestyle can further exacerbate these conditions. As a result, managing inflammation is essential not only for immediate symptom relief but also for preventing age-related diseases that can substantially effect quality of life. Women over 60 are particularly vulnerable to inflammation due to the compounding effects of aging and hormonal changes. The post-menopausal body experiences shifts in bone density, muscle mass, and fat distribution, and this can result in a rise in the storage of fat, particularly visceral fat around the abdominal region. This type of fat is highly inflammatory and contributes to the release of pro-inflammatory cytokines, molecules that perpetuate the cycle of inflammation. Visceral fat is also linked to insulin resistance, raising the risk for type 2 diabetes—a condition that has a direct connection to chronic inflammation. Moreover, the cardiovascular system also undergoes significant changes with age. Arterial stiffness, high blood pressure, and the buildup of plaque in the arteries are all associated with chronic inflammation. In older women, heart disease is the main cause of mortality, and these changes raise the chance of developing heart disease. There is also a significant contribution that inflammation makes to the onset of osteoporosis, a condition marked by a decrease in bone density that disproportionately affects post-menopausal women. The loss of bone mass is frequently followed by inflammation in the joints, which could result in disorders like osteoarthritis, which may bring about pain, stiffness, and a reduction in mobility. Addressing inflammation in women over 60 is not just about managing symptoms— adopting a preventative perspective to health that encourages a graceful ageing process is the focus of this concept. Diet plays a pivotal role in this process. An anti-inflammatory diet, rich in whole, nutrient-dense foods, can help combat the negative effects of aging and reduce inflammation throughout the body. By prioritizing foods that are known to lower inflammation and avoiding those that contribute to it, women can take control of their health, support their immune system, and enhance their longevity.

Chapter 1: Understanding Body Changes After 60

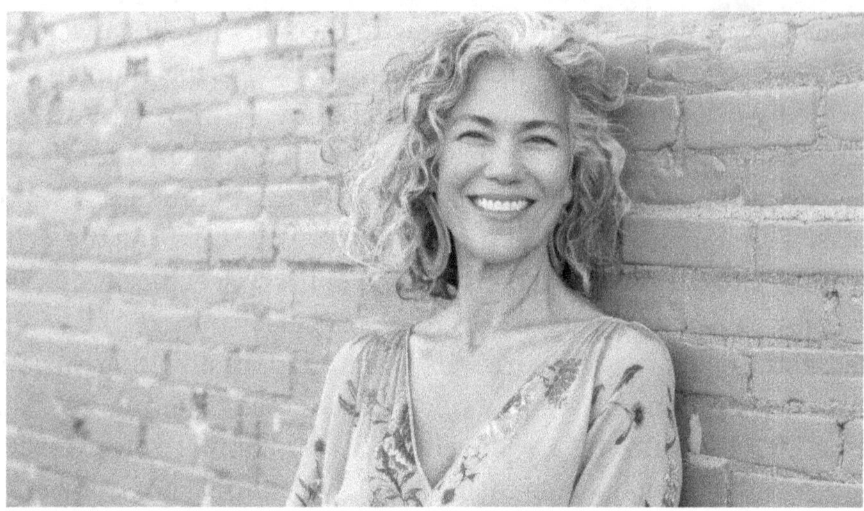

As women enter their 60s, their bodies undergo significant changes that can affect both physical and emotional well-being. These changes, largely driven by hormonal shifts, aging, and lifestyle factors, manifest in various systems, from bone and cardiovascular health to cognitive function. During this period of life, it is crucial to have a thorough comprehension of these modifications in order to make well-informed decisions that will enhance health and longevity.

1.1 Menopause and Hormonal Changes

Menopause is a defining transition for women as they age, typically occurring in the late 40s to early 50s, but its effects are long-lasting. The hallmark of menopause is the significant decline in estrogen and progesterone production, two hormones essential for reproductive function and overall health. After menopause, women experience a range of changes due to the reduced presence of these hormones. The hormone estrogen, in specific, is responsible for providing protection to a variety of the body's systems. Its decline contributes to a higher risk of chronic inflammation, it has the potential to result in a wide range of age-related diseases. The anti-inflammatory impacts of estrogen help protect against diseases like heart disease, osteoporosis, and even some neurodegenerative conditions. With less estrogen, women over 60 are more prone to experiencing joint pain, stiffness, and other inflammatory issues. Additionally, this hormonal drop impacts the skin, leading to thinning, dryness, and a reduction in elasticity, contributing to the visible signs of aging. Another key area affected by menopause is fat distribution. Instead of accumulating fat around the hips and thighs, fat tends to collect around the belly as a result of the hormonal shift that occurs during menopause. A higher risk of metabolic syndrome, type 2 diabetes, and cardiovascular disease has been associated with visceral fat, which is a form of fat that is found in the abdominal cavity. As a result, weight management becomes a challenge, often requiring adjustments to diet and physical activity to maintain a healthy weight.

1.2 Bone Health and Osteoporosis

One of the most critical effects of post-menopausal hormonal changes is the effect on bone health. Estrogen is essential for preserving bone density, and after menopause, women experience accelerated bone loss, which increases their risk of osteoporosis. Osteoporosis is a condition where bones become brittle and more susceptible to fractures, particularly in the spine, hips, and wrists. After menopause, people have a considerable slowdown in the process of bone remodeling, which is the process by which old bone tissue is substituted by new bone. As a result, bone density decreases at a faster rate, especially in the first few years following menopause. By the time women reach their 60s, many are at an elevated risk of experiencing fractures from falls or even minor impacts. This increased fragility can greatly affect mobility and independence, leading to longer recovery times and a potential loss of quality of life. It is crucial for women over the age of 60 to be certain that they are consuming sufficient quantities of calcium, vitamin D, and other minerals that are critical to bone strength in order to achieve and maintain bone health. Weight-bearing exercises, such as walking, strength training, and yoga, can also help maintain bone density and improve balance, reducing the risk of falls. Hormonal replacement therapies or other medications may be considered under medical supervision to slow down bone loss for women at high risk of osteoporosis.

1.3 Cardiovascular Health

Cardiovascular health is another area significantly impacted by the aging process, especially in women over 60. Estrogen has a protective effect on the heart and blood vessels, helping to regulate cholesterol levels and maintain the elasticity of arteries. After menopause, women experience an increase in LDL (bad) cholesterol and a decrease in HDL (good) cholesterol. It is possible that this shift could result in the accumulation of plaque in the arteries, which will in turn increase the risk of atherosclerosis, cardiovascular disease, and stroke. The decline in estrogen also contributes to increased arterial stiffness, which raises blood pressure. Hypertension, or high blood pressure, becomes more common in women over 60 and is a major contributor to the development of cardiovascular disease. Without estrogen's protective influence, women's cardiovascular risk factors become more like those of men, making it critical to manage cholesterol levels, blood pressure, and other heart health indicators through diet, exercise, and sometimes medication. The importance of physical activity cannot be overstated when it comes to the maintenance of cardiovascular health. Participating in regular physical activity not only assists in weight management but also serves to improve circulation, strengthen the heart muscle, and assist in the management of blood pressure. The risk of cardiovascular disease can be considerably reduced by following a diet that is heart-healthy, anti-inflammatory, and abundant in fruits, vegetables, whole grains, and healthy fats like omega-3 fatty acids.

1.4 Cognitive Changes

The brain, like the rest of the body, undergoes changes as women age. While not all women experience cognitive decline after 60, some may notice memory lapses, difficulty concentrating, or slower cognitive processing. These changes can be linked to hormonal shifts, particularly the reduction of estrogen, which affects brain function. The reduction of estrogen has been linked to a greater likelihood of neurodegenerative disorders such as Alzheimer's disease. Estrogen plays a function in shielding the brain from inflammation and oxidative stress, and its low levels have been related with this risk. It is more common for women who have gone through menopause to get Alzheimer's disease than it is for men of the same age, making brain health a critical focus for women over 60. A poor diet, a lack of physical activity, and persistent stress are all examples of lifestyle factors that can lead to cognitive alterations. Hormonal issues are also a potential contributor to these changes. High levels of stress, in particular, can increase the production of cortisol, a hormone that negatively impacts memory and learning over time. Sleep disturbances, often common after menopause, can further contribute to cognitive challenges, because a good night's sleep is necessary for the consolidation of memories and the general health of the brain. Maintaining cognitive health involves staying mentally active through continuous learning, social engagement, and brain-challenging activities like puzzles, reading, and problem-solving. A nutrient-rich diet that supports brain health, involving foods rich in antioxidants and omega-3 fatty acids, along with regular physical exercise, can also help preserve cognitive function as women age.

1.5 Other Effects of Aging

Beyond the significant changes to bone health, cardiovascular function, and cognitive abilities, aging brings about a variety of other physiological effects that can effect a woman's overall health and quality of life. One of the most prominent changes is the slowing down of metabolism. After 60, the body becomes less efficient at burning calories, which can lead to gradual weight gain, especially when combined with reduced physical activity. This decline in metabolic rate is often accompanied by the loss of muscle mass, a condition known as sarcopenia. As muscles naturally shrink with age, women may notice a decrease in strength, endurance, and energy levels. This reduction in muscle mass not only affects physical capabilities but also contributes to a slower metabolism, creating a cycle that can make weight management more challenging. Incorporating strength-training exercises can help counteract these effects, preserving muscle and boosting metabolic health. Joint health also becomes a growing concern as women age. It is possible for disorders such as osteoarthritis to develop as a result of the wear and strain that occurs on joints over time, notably in the knees, hips, and hands. Stiffness, soreness, and decreased mobility are among symptoms that can result from the wear and tear of the cartilage that cushions the joints. Maintaining flexibility and joint function through low-impact exercises such as yoga, swimming, and gentle stretching is crucial to preserving mobility and preventing injury.

In addition to joint issues, women may also experience a decline in balance, hence elevating the likelihood of experiencing fractures and falls, further highlighting the importance of regular physical activity and balance training.

Vision and eye health are also affected by the aging process. Many women, after the age of sixty, face changes in their vision. Some of the most prevalent concerns are cataracts, age-related macular degeneration (AMD), and presbyopia, which is characterized by trouble concentrating on objects that are close to the eye. These conditions can significantly impair day-to-day activities like reading, driving, and recognizing faces. Regular eye exams, along with a diet rich in antioxidants, particularly lutein and zeaxanthin found in leafy greens, can support eye health and help slow the progression of vision problems. Similarly, hearing loss is another sensory change that can occur with age, impacting communication and social engagement.

Digestive health often becomes more sensitive as well. Constipation, bloating, and discomfort are some of the concerns that might arise as a result of the slowing metabolism of the digestive system. The efficiency of nutrient absorption may also decline, making it essential to prioritize foods that are nutrient-dense and high in fiber. Probiotics and prebiotics, found in fermented foods and certain supplements, can support a healthy gut microbiome, which is critical for digestive health, immune function, and overall well-being.

Lastly, the immune system weakens as women age, a phenomenon known as immunosenescence. The body becomes more prone to infections, diseases, and a delayed recovery from injuries as a result of this loss in immunological function. Supporting the immune system through a balanced diet rich in vitamins and minerals, regular exercise, proper sleep, and stress management can help boost the body's defenses. Hydration also plays a crucial role, as older adults are more prone to dehydration, which can affect energy levels, cognition, and overall bodily function.

Chapter 2: What Is The Anti-Inflammatory Diet?

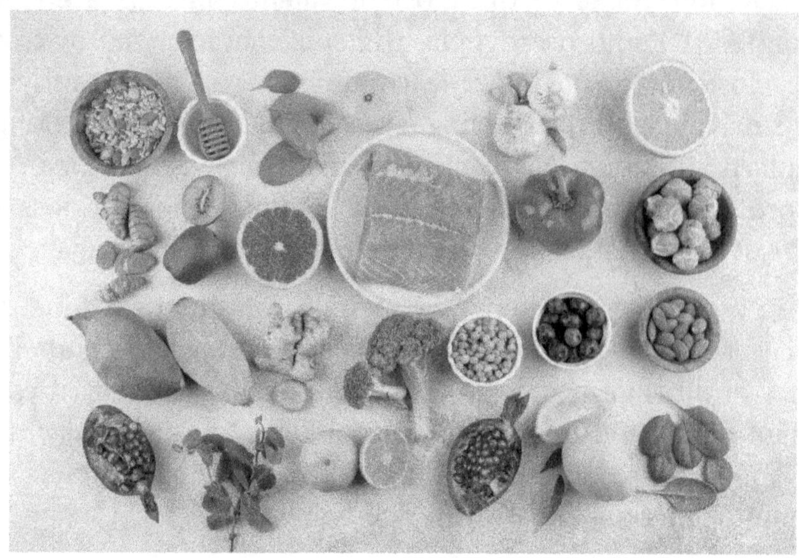

2.1 Understanding Inflammation: Causes and Effects

Inflammation is a response that occurs naturally and is required by the immune system of the body in response to an injury, an infection, or even damaging stimuli. It is a protective mechanism designed to heal wounds, fight off infections, and respond to toxins or irritants. When the body detects a threat—whether it's a cut, a bacterial infection, or exposure to harmful substances—white blood cells and other immune components rush to the site to contain the damage and begin the healing process. This response is known as **acute inflammation**, and it is distinguished by redness, swelling, heat, and discomfort accompanied by these symptoms. In the short term, acute inflammation is beneficial and vital for survival, as it helps the body recover from various injuries and infections.

Nevertheless, not all forms of inflammation are beneficial. **Chronic inflammation** is a condition that can last for several months or even long years, occurs when the inflammatory response becomes misdirected or fails to shut down properly. Instead of resolving, the inflammation lingers and becomes a constant, low-level presence in the body. Unlike acute inflammation, which is temporary and focused on a specific area, chronic inflammation can be widespread and affect multiple systems at once. This type of prolonged inflammation can gradually damage tissues and organs, leading to a host of chronic diseases. There are several potential **causes** of chronic inflammation. One major factor is **lifestyle-related**: poor diet, lack of exercise, chronic stress, and insufficient sleep can all contribute to ongoing inflammatory responses. For example, a diet that is high in processed foods, sweets, and unhealthy fats might encourage the synthesis of chemicals that are associated with inflammation in the cardiovascular system. Similarly, a sedentary lifestyle can lead to obesity, which is itself a major driver of inflammation. Adipose tissue, particularly the visceral fat stored around the abdomen, releases inflammatory substances that can worsen systemic inflammation.

Another key cause of chronic inflammation is **environmental exposure** to toxins, pollutants, and irritants. Air pollution, chemical exposure, and cigarette smoke are all examples of environmental factors that can trigger inflammation. In some cases, the body's immune system may continuously react to these irritants, leading to a cycle of ongoing inflammation. Chronic infections or **autoimmune diseases** are also common causes. Rheumatoid arthritis, lupus, and multiple sclerosis are examples of autoimmune disorders that manifest themselves when the immune system wrongly targets the tissues of the body, leading to long-term inflammation and tissue damage. Chronic infections, such as those caused by viruses, bacteria, or fungi that the body cannot fully eliminate, can also lead to persistent inflammation. The **effects** of chronic inflammation are widespread and often subtle at first, making it difficult to detect until more severe health problems arise. Chronic inflammation has the potential to play a role in the emergence of a wide variety of serious health disorders since it persists over time. For example, one of the most well-documented effects of chronic inflammation is its role in **cardiovascular disease**. There is a correlation between chronic inflammation and the development of atherosclerosis, which is characterized by the accumulation of fatty plaques in the arteries, which in turn raises the risk of cardiovascular events like heart attacks and strokes. Inflammatory markers, like C-reactive protein (CRP), are frequently increased in persons who suffer from heart disease.

Chronic inflammation is also closely linked to **type 2 diabetes**. When inflammatory molecules are present, they hinder the body's capacity to make effective utilization of insulin, which ultimately results in insulin resistance, which is a precursor to diabetes. Once diabetes is established, high blood sugar levels can further fuel inflammation, creating a vicious cycle that exacerbates both conditions. **Obesity**, particularly when associated with high levels of visceral fat, is another condition where inflammation plays a central role, as adipose tissue itself releases inflammatory signals that affect the whole body. In the case of **neurodegenerative diseases** like Alzheimer's and Parkinson's, inflammation has been shown to contribute to the progressive damage and loss of brain cells. There is a correlation between Alzheimer's disease and the accumulation of toxic proteins, like amyloid plaques, which can be accelerated by chronic inflammation in the brain. This process is often mentioned to as **neuroinflammation**, and it plays a significant role in cognitive decline and other age-related neurological disorders.

Another significant effect of chronic inflammation is its role in the enhancement of **cancer**. Inflammation is a natural aspect of the body's defense mechanism; however, if it continues for an extended period of time, it can cause damage to DNA and encourage the growth and survival of aberrant cells, which can ultimately result in the development of tumors. Certain cancers, like colon, liver, and pancreatic cancers, have been closely associated with chronic inflammation, particularly in individuals with inflammatory bowel disease, hepatitis, or other conditions where inflammation persists over long periods.

Finally, chronic inflammation plays a key role in **joint health**, particularly in conditions like arthritis. **Osteoarthritis**, although traditionally seen as a "wear and tear" disease, is now understood to have an inflammatory component. The breakdown of cartilage in the joints can trigger a low-grade inflammatory response that worsens the condition over time.

Rheumatoid arthritis, an autoimmune condition, involves a much more aggressive inflammatory process, where the immune system directly attacks joint tissues, leading to pain, swelling, and deformity.

In conclusion, while inflammation is a necessary and beneficial process when it comes to acute injury or infection, chronic inflammation is a different story. When left unchecked, it can silently fuel the development of many serious health conditions, ranging from cardiovascular disease and diabetes to neurodegenerative disorders and cancer. Understanding the causes of chronic inflammation, from lifestyle factors to environmental exposures and underlying medical conditions, is crucial for identifying ways to reduce inflammation and protect long-term health.

2.2 Benefits of Reducing Inflammation

Reducing inflammation in the body is not just about addressing the immediate symptoms of pain, swelling, or discomfort. It's about tackling an underlying issue that can have profound, long-term advantages for one's health and well-being that are comprehensive. By minimizing chronic inflammation, individuals can protect themselves from a host of serious health conditions that are closely linked to ongoing inflammatory processes. The avoidance of **cardiovascular diseases** is one of the biggest advantages that can be gained from lowering inflammation. The accumulation of plaque in the arteries, which causes the arteries to become narrower and increases the risk of heart attacks and strokes, is a condition known as atherosclerosis. Chronic inflammation plays a significant role in the progression of atherosclerosis. When inflammation is kept under control, it helps to stabilize these plaques and reduce the likelihood of dangerous cardiovascular events. Another major benefit is the **improvement in metabolic health**. Chronic inflammation is a key driver of insulin resistance, which can lead to type 2 diabetes. Lowering inflammation makes the body more susceptible to insulin, which in turn makes it possible for glucose to be processed more effectively and brings to a reduction in their blood sugar levels. This can help avoid or manage diabetes and its related complications. Additionally, controlling inflammation helps with weight management. Since inflammation and obesity are closely linked—particularly through visceral fat—reducing inflammation can make it easier to lose weight and maintain a healthy metabolism. For those with **autoimmune diseases** like rheumatoid arthritis or lupus, reducing inflammation can significantly improve quality of life. In autoimmune disorders, the immune system attacks the body's own tissues, which is a characteristic feature of these diseases, resulting in painful and debilitating inflammation. By managing and lowering inflammation, individuals can experience fewer flare-ups, reduced pain, and less damage to joints, skin, and other organs. This can slow the progression of the disease and lead to improved mobility, function, and overall well-being.

Reducing inflammation also has profound effects on **brain health**. Neuroinflammation, or inflammation within the brain, cognitive decline and neurodegenerative disorders such as Alzheimer's disease have been related to neurodegenerative conditions. By keeping inflammation in check, individuals may protect their cognitive functions, improve memory, and lower the risk of developing dementia or other age-related cognitive disorders.

Lowering inflammation may also help with mood regulation and reduce symptoms of depression and anxiety, which have been linked to chronic inflammation in recent research.

For those struggling with **joint health**, particularly with conditions like osteoarthritis or rheumatoid arthritis, reducing inflammation can alleviate joint pain, stiffness, and swelling. This, in turn, can improve mobility, allowing individuals to stay active and maintain their independence as they age. Physical activity is key to managing both inflammation and overall health, and reduced joint inflammation makes staying active more comfortable and sustainable. Additionally, reducing inflammation has been linked to **cancer prevention**. Chronic inflammation can cause DNA damage and increase the formation of aberrant cells, both of which can contribute to the development of some malignancies. Inflammation naturally occurs as a component of the immune response of the body; however, chronic inflammation can be harmful. By minimizing inflammation, individuals can lower the risk of cancers that are linked with chronic inflammatory conditions, like colon, liver, and pancreatic cancer. Finally, lowering inflammation can support a **stronger immune system**. It is possible for chronic inflammation to impair the immune system, which in turn makes the body more vulnerable to infections, viruses, and diseases. By lowering this persistent inflammation, the immune system can function more effectively, improving overall resilience to disease and ensuring quicker recovery from illness.

The cumulative effect of reducing chronic inflammation is a longer, healthier life, with reduced risk for serious diseases and improved day-to-day functioning. Whether through dietary changes, exercise, stress management, or other lifestyle modifications, when it comes to protecting and improving one's health over the long term, one of the most effective methods is to actively reduce inflammation.

2.3 The Role of Diet in Managing Inflammation

Inflammation in the body can be managed and reduced to a significant extent through the use of diet. The foods we eat have a direct effect on the levels of inflammatory markers in our system, and the right dietary choices can significantly lower chronic inflammation. Conversely, poor dietary habits can exacerbate inflammation and aid to the advancement of various health issues. Realizing the connection between diet and inflammation is essential for adopting an anti-inflammatory lifestyle and preventing the onset of related diseases. One of the most important ways in which diet can affect inflammation is by ensuring that there is a healthy mix of foods that are both **pro-inflammatory** and **anti-inflammatory**. Inflammatory meals, also known as pro-inflammatory foods, are typically highly processed, high in added sugars, refined carbs, and unhealthy fats. These foods are also known to induce inflammation in the body. For example, foods like sugary snacks, white bread, fried foods, and processed meats are known to promote the production of inflammatory molecules such as cytokines. Additionally, trans fats and excessive omega-6 fatty acids, commonly found in fast foods and processed snacks, can disturb the body's natural balance of fatty acids, triggering inflammatory responses. On the other hand, anti-inflammatory foods contain **nutrients and compounds** that actively fight inflammation and promote healing. **Omega-3 fatty acids** are considered to be one of the best-known elements of an anti-inflammatory diet.

These acids can be found in fatty fish like salmon, mackerel, and sardines, as well as in flaxseeds and walnuts. Omega-3 fatty acids are extremely effective at lowering the levels of pro-inflammatory markers in the body and also assist in restoring a healthy balance to the omega-6 fatty acids that are present in a variety of processed meals. It is possible for individuals to reduce inflammation, enhance heart health, and protect themselves against neurodegenerative illnesses by elevating their consumption of omega-3 fatty acids.

Another key element of an anti-inflammatory diet is the inclusion of **antioxidant-rich foods**, particularly fruits and vegetables. The presence of free radicals, which are molecules that are unstable and lead to oxidative stress and inflammation, can be neutralized with the assistance of antioxidants. Berries, leafy greens, bell peppers, and tomatoes are just a few of the colorful fruits and vegetables that are loaded with vitamins, minerals, and antioxidants such as vitamins C and E, flavonoids, and carotenoids. These nutrients not only contribute to the reduction of inflammation, but they also help to strengthen the immune system and improve your general well-being.

Whole grains, like brown rice, quinoa, and oats, also play a crucial role in managing inflammation. Unlike refined grains, which can spike blood sugar and contribute to inflammation, in addition to promoting good digestion and helping to maintain normal blood sugar levels, whole grains include a high amount of fiber. Additionally, fiber helps to maintain a healthy microbiome in the gut, which is becoming more widely recognized as an important element in the regulation of inflammation. A balanced gut microbiome can reduce systemic inflammation and support better digestion and immune function.

In addition to specific foods, there are also **herbs and spices** known for their anti-inflammatory properties. Turmeric, which contains the active compound curcumin, is particularly powerful in reducing inflammation. Ginger, garlic, cinnamon, and green tea are other natural anti-inflammatory agents that can be easily incorporated into meals. Not only can these meals improve flavour, but they also help to a healthier and better balanced inflammatory response. Equally important to managing inflammation through diet is the **avoidance of foods** that trigger or worsen inflammation. Because they encourage inflammation and are linked to weight gain, insulin resistance, and other chronic illnesses, processed foods, sugary snacks, and refined carbs should be minimized. This is because they are examples of foods that lead to inflammation. Similarly, alcohol and excessive caffeine intake can provoke inflammatory responses and should be consumed in moderation.

Overall, adopting an anti-inflammatory diet involves making conscious choices to include nutrient-dense, whole foods that support the body's natural ability to fight inflammation, while avoiding processed and inflammatory-triggering foods. The role of diet in managing inflammation is not just about preventing disease but about actively promoting longevity, vitality, and overall health.

Chapter 3: Types of Anti-Inflammatory Diets

3.1 Mediterranean Diet

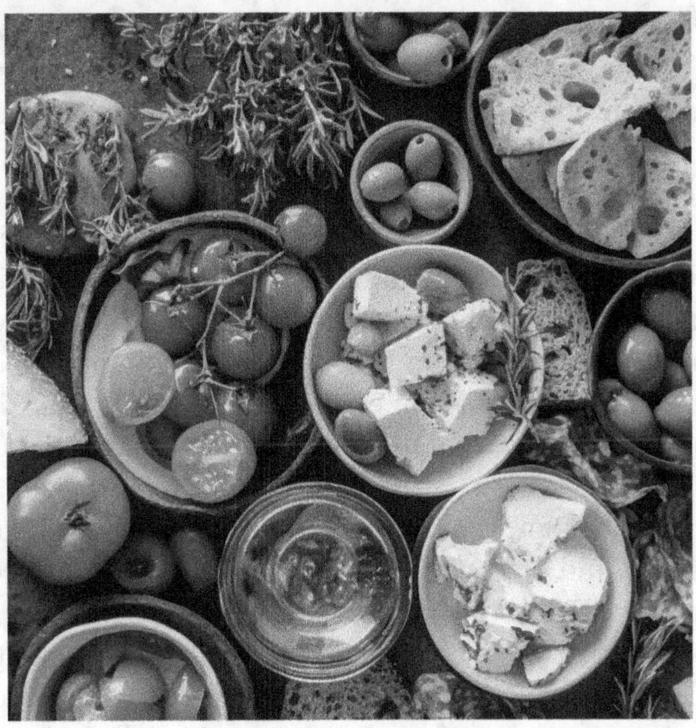

Due in large part to the significant anti-inflammatory benefits that it possesses, the Mediterranean diet is one of the dietary patterns that has been the subject of the most extensive research and is frequently advocated for the purpose of increasing health and longevity. This diet depends on the traditional eating practices of nations that border the Mediterranean Sea, like Greece, Italy, and Spain, and it places an emphasis on whole foods, minimally processed foods that are naturally rich in anti-inflammatory compounds. The Mediterranean diet is not just a meal plan but a lifestyle, incorporating a balanced approach to eating that is both enjoyable and sustainable. In the Mediterranean diet, the consumption of **healthy fats**, specifically **olive oil**, which is used in a substantial amount in both cooking and dressing, is the most important component. Olive oil, particularly extra-virgin olive oil, is not only abundant in monounsaturated fats but also includes polyphenols, which are known to possess powerful anti-inflammatory and antioxidant properties. Inflammation in the body can be prevented with the aid of these chemicals, protect the cardiovascular system, and support overall cellular health. In addition to olive oil, other healthy fat sources such as **nuts**, **seeds**, and **fatty fish** like salmon, sardines, and mackerel are key components. These fish are rich in omega-3 fatty acids, which are known to lower inflammatory markers and enhance heart health. One of the most important aspects of the Mediterranean diet is the value placed on meals that are derived from plants. On a daily basis, a broad range of fruits and vegetables are consumed, which results in the consumption of a substantial quantity of vitamins, minerals, essential fiber, and antioxidants.

These nutrients contribute to the reduction of oxidative stress, the neutralization of free radicals, and the reduction of inflammation. Leafy greens, tomatoes, peppers, and cruciferous vegetables like broccoli and cauliflower are staples in this diet, offering a broad spectrum of protective compounds. Fruits such as berries, citrus, and pomegranates are particularly valued for their high antioxidant content. Another essential element of the Mediterranean diet is the consumption of whole grains. These grains include **whole wheat, brown rice, quinoa,** and **barley** are examples. These grains include a high amount of fiber, which is beneficial to digestive health and assists to maintain healthy blood sugar levels, and promotes a balanced gut microbiome—all of which contribute to reduced inflammation. Unlike refined grains that can spike blood sugar and trigger inflammatory responses, whole grains are absorbed more slowly, providing sustained energy and stabilizing blood sugar levels. Within the context of the Mediterranean diet, **legumes**, which include beans, lentils, and chickpeas, constitute an essential source of plant-based protein and various types of fiber. These foods are low in fat and high in complex carbohydrates, making them an excellent option for supporting heart health and reducing inflammation. In addition to legumes, moderate amounts of **dairy**, especially in the form of cheese and yoghurt, are incorporated into this diet. These foods provide a source of calcium as well as probiotics, which are beneficial to the health of the gut. One of the key aspects of the Mediterranean diet is its approach to **protein sources**. While fish is the primary animal protein consumed, **poultry** and **eggs** are eaten in moderation, while **red meat** is limited to only occasional consumption. This shift away from red meat, which is often associated with higher levels of inflammation, contributes to the diet's anti-inflammatory benefits. Instead, plant-based proteins from legumes and nuts are emphasized. The Mediterranean diet also includes **moderate consumption of red wine**, especially when it comes to eating. **Resveratrol** is a molecule that may be found in the skin of grapes and is known to have anti-inflammatory and antioxidant activities. Red wine includes resveratrol. On the other hand, moderation is essential, as drinking a great deal of alcohol can have a reverse impact and perhaps contribute to a rise in inflammation. In general, the Mediterranean diet is a dietary pattern that is nutrient-dense, well-balanced, and places an emphasis on whole foods, healthy fats, and nutrients that are derived from plants. Its emphasis on anti-inflammatory nutrients and avoidance of processed, pro-inflammatory foods makes it an ideal choice for reducing chronic inflammation and promoting long-term health.

3.2 DASH Diet

The **DASH diet**, which stands for the Dietary Approaches to Stop Hypertension, was initially intended to assist individuals in the management of high blood pressure. However, it has subsequently earned recognition for its wider range of health advantages, including its capacity to lower inflammation. Whole, nutrient-dense foods are the primary focus of the DASH diet, which is designed to promote heart health, lower oxidative stress, and reduce the likelihood of developing chronic inflammation. Like the Mediterranean diet, it encourages the consumption of foods that are naturally anti-inflammatory while limiting those that can contribute to inflammation.

At the heart of the DASH diet is its emphasis on **fruits and vegetables**, which are rich in vitamins, minerals, fiber, and antioxidants. By including a wide diversity of colorful produce, like berries, leafy greens, cruciferous vegetables, and citrus fruits, the DASH diet provides a wealth of nutrients that help reduce inflammation. These foods are particularly high in potassium, magnesium, and calcium, which play a critical role in regulating blood pressure and promoting cardiovascular health. Potassium, in particular, helps to balance sodium levels in the body, which could ease water retention and lower blood pressure, while also supporting the body's inflammatory response. In addition to fruits and vegetables, the DASH diet emphasizes the consumption of **whole grains**. Whole grains like brown rice, quinoa, oats, and whole wheat bread are a significant source of fiber, which helps to regulate digestion, control blood sugar levels, and support a healthy gut microbiome. These grains are absorbed more slowly than refined grains, preventing the blood sugar spikes that can trigger inflammation. Fiber is also vital to keeping a healthy weight, which is essential because extra fat in the body can lead to a variety of health problems, particularly visceral fat, is a known contributor to chronic inflammation. The DASH diet also promotes **lean proteins**, such as **poultry**, **fish**, and **plant-based proteins** like beans and lentils. Compared to red meat, these types of protein offer a smaller amount of saturated fats, which can be a factor in inflammation. Additionally, these sources of protein supply important amino acids, which are beneficial for maintaining muscle growth and overall body function. Fish particularly is recommended because of the omega-3 fatty acids that it contains. These acids have been demonstrated to decrease inflammation and to support the health of the heart. While the DASH diet allows for some animal protein, it advises limiting red meat and processed meats, which are associated with higher levels of inflammatory markers in the body. **Low-fat dairy products**, such as yogurt, milk, and cheese, are another key component of the DASH diet. These foods provide calcium and vitamin D, which are important for bone health and can help reduce inflammation in the body. Probiotic-rich yogurt, in particular, can also support gut health by promoting a balanced microbiome, which is increasingly recognized as an important factor in controlling inflammation. The DASH diet is also low in **sodium**. The consumption of a high amount of sodium is linked to elevated blood pressure and has the potential to worsen inflammation, especially for individuals who are reactive to and susceptible to salt. By favoring fresh, natural meals and minimizing the use of processed foods that are high in sodium, the DASH diet helps to reduce water retention, improve blood vessel function, and lower overall inflammation levels. Another important aspect of the DASH diet is its limitation of **added sugars and unhealthy fats**. Processed foods, sugary snacks, and beverages high in refined sugars are avoided, as they can cause blood sugar spikes, insulin resistance, and increased inflammatory responses. Instead, healthy fats, such as those found in nuts, seeds, and avocados, are included in moderation. These fats, along with the polyunsaturated and monounsaturated fats found in fish and olive oil, help to lower bad cholesterol and reduce inflammation.

Overall, the DASH diet is designed to promote heart health, control blood pressure, and reduce chronic inflammation through a balanced approach to nutrition. By emphasizing nutrient-dense, whole foods while limiting processed and pro-inflammatory ingredients, the DASH diet provides a sustainable way to support long-term health and well-being.

3.3 Plant-Based Diets

Plant-based diets have gained widespread recognition for their numerous health benefits, particularly when it comes to decreasing inflammation. These diets prioritize whole, minimally processed plant foods while limiting or completely avoiding animal products. Although the degree to which animal products are restricted can vary, plant-based diets generally focus on fruits, vegetables, whole grains, legumes, nuts, and seeds as the primary sources of nutrients. The anti-inflammatory effects of plant-based diets stem from the abundance of antioxidants, fiber, and healthy fats found in these foods, as well as the reduction in saturated fats and pro-inflammatory compounds often present in animal-based products. **Antioxidants** are found in high concentrations in plant-based diets, which is one of the fundamental advantages of these diets. There is a high concentration of vitamins, minerals, and phytonutrients in fruits and vegetables, which contribute to the neutralization of free radicals and the reduction of oxidative stress in the body. By lowering oxidative stress, plant-based diets can help to decrease the chronic inflammation that contributes to numerous diseases, involving heart disease, diabetes, and certain cancers. Leafy greens, berries, cruciferous vegetables, and brightly colored fruits and vegetables are especially powerful in this regard, offering a wide range of antioxidants such as vitamin C, vitamin E, flavonoids, and carotenoids. Another significant component of plant-based diets is **fiber**. Fiber is an essential component in maintaining healthy gut function, which is increasingly recognized as a key factor in managing inflammation. A healthy gut microbiome, which is fostered by fiber-rich foods, can help regulate immune responses and reduce systemic inflammation. Plant-based diets, which are naturally high in fiber from fruits, vegetables, legumes, and whole grains, promote healthy digestion, stabilize blood sugar levels, and support a balanced gut microbiome. This, in turn, helps reduce the risk of inflammatory conditions such as obesity, type 2 diabetes, and metabolic syndrome.

Additionally, to antioxidants and fiber, **healthy fats** from plant sources contribute to the anti-inflammatory effects of plant-based diets. Foods such as avocados, almonds, seeds, and olive oil are examples of foods that include monounsaturated and polyunsaturated compounds, which are known to reduce inflammation and improve cardiovascular health. In instance, flaxseeds, chia seeds, and walnuts are rich sources of omega-3 fatty acids, which are vital in reducing inflammatory indicators in the body. Flaxseeds are also a good source of omega-6 fatty acids. By prioritizing these healthy fats and reducing the intake of saturated fats found in animal products, plant-based diets help to support overall health and decrease the risk of chronic inflammatory diseases. An essential aspect of plant-based diets is the **exclusion or limitation of animal products**, particularly red and processed meats. In addition to being associated with a higher likelihood of cardiovascular disease, cancer, and other chronic illnesses, these meats frequently include a high amount of saturated fats, which can lead to a rise in inflammation.

By substituting these items with plant-based proteins like quinoa, tofu, tempeh, and lentils, we can reduce our protein intake, individuals following plant-based diets can benefit from lower levels of inflammatory markers and improved overall health. One further advantage of plant-based diets is their capacity to facilitate the management of weight in a healthy manner. With plant-based diets, which are often lower in calories and higher in nutritional density, individuals are able to sustain a healthy weight.

Obesity is a primary driver of chronic inflammation, and plant-based diets may assist individuals attain and keep a healthy weight. By reducing excess body fat, particularly visceral fat, plant-based diets can significantly lower inflammation levels and decrease the likelihood of obesity-related diseases.

Overall, plant-based diets offer a holistic approach to reducing inflammation and improving long-term health. By focusing on nutrient-dense, whole plant foods and minimizing or eliminating pro-inflammatory animal products, these diets complement the natural anti-inflammatory processes that occur within the body in a way that is both sustainable and effective.

3.4 Low-Glycemic Diets

Low-glycemic diets are another highly effective dietary approach for managing inflammation and promoting overall health. These diets focus on foods that have a low glycemic index (GI), which means they are digested and absorbed more slowly, causing a gradual rise in blood sugar levels rather than a sharp spike. By avoiding high-glycemic foods that cause rapid increases in blood sugar, low-glycemic diets help to stabilize insulin levels, reduce inflammation, and prevent the development of chronic conditions like diabetes and cardiovascular disease.

One of the main mechanisms through which low-glycemic diets reduce inflammation is by **preventing blood sugar spikes**. The consumption of foods that are high in glycemic index, like white bread, sugary snacks, and refined carbs, leads to a rise in the synthesis of insulin, which in turn causes fast spikes in blood glucose levels. This can, eventually, develop in insulin resistance, which is a condition in which the cells of the body become less receptive to insulin. This condition leads to persistently high levels of blood sugar as well as increased inflammation. Individuals are able to preserve more stable blood sugar levels and lower the inflammatory responses that are linked with insulin resistance if they choose foods that have a low glycemic index. Some examples of these foods are legumes, whole grains, vegetables that are not starchy, and some fruits.

Another important aspect of low-glycemic diets is their emphasis on **whole, unprocessed foods**. Many of the foods that are low on the glycemic index are also rich in fiber, vitamins, minerals, and antioxidants, all of which aid to lower inflammation levels. Whole grains, such as oats, quinoa, and barley, are absorbed more slowly than refined grains, providing sustained energy and helping to prevent the blood sugar fluctuations that can trigger inflammatory responses. Not only are non-starchy veggies like broccoli, spinach, and peppers low in calories, but they also have a low glycemic load, which makes them good choices for preserving stable blood sugar levels and lowering inflammation. The use of **legumes**, which include beans, lentils, and chickpeas, represents a fundamental component of low-glycemic diets and offers a multitude of advantages to one's health. Not only are these meals low on the glycemic index, but they are also high in protein and fiber, both of which contribute to the regulation of digestion and the maintenance of better gut health, and promote stable blood sugar levels. By incorporating legumes into meals, individuals can enjoy a satisfying source of plant-based protein that helps to reduce inflammation and support long-term metabolic health.

Low-glycemic diets also prioritize **healthy fats** from sources like nuts, seeds, avocados, and olive oil. These fats, particularly omega-3 fatty acids, help to reduce inflammation and support cardiovascular health. Since high-glycemic diets are often associated with increased levels of harmful fats, like trans fats and excessive saturated fats, low-glycemic diets offer a more heart-healthy approach by focusing on beneficial fats that support overall health.

In addition to choosing low-glycemic foods, it is essential to **avoid high-glycemic foods**, which can contribute to chronic inflammation. Refined sugars, white bread, pastries, and sugary drinks are some of the worst offenders, due to the fact that they produce sudden spikes in blood sugar and cause inflammatory processes to be triggered within the body. These foods are often devoid of the fiber and nutrients needed to support stable blood sugar levels and can lead to weight gain, insulin resistance, and increased risk of diabetes. Low-glycemic diets can also help with **weight management**, another critical factor in reducing inflammation. By focusing on foods that provide sustained energy and promote feelings of fullness, diets that are low in glycemic index can assist persons in maintaining a healthy weight, hence lowering the risk of inflammation that is associated with obesity. Maintaining a healthy weight is essential for reducing inflammation in the body, as excess fat, particularly around the abdomen, is a major source of inflammatory cytokines.

In summary, low-glycemic diets offer a powerful way to reduce inflammation by promoting stable blood sugar levels, supporting metabolic health, and reducing the intake of pro-inflammatory foods. By focusing on whole, nutrient-dense foods with a low glycemic index, individuals can protect themselves from chronic inflammation and improve overall well-being.

3.5 Empowering Women Over 60: Navigating the Anti-Inflammatory Diet

For women over 60, adopting an anti-inflammatory diet can be a transformative step towards improving overall health and well-being. As the body undergoes various changes with age, including hormonal shifts and increased susceptibility to chronic conditions, selecting the right dietary approach becomes essential. One beneficial strategy is the incorporation of intermittent fasting, which has gained popularity for its ability to reduce inflammatory markers and enhance metabolic health. This approach involves alternating periods of eating with periods of fasting, allowing the body to enter a state of autophagy, where it cleanses and repairs cells, potentially lowering inflammation. In the process of deciding what to eat, women of this age should prioritize consuming foods that are high in nutrients and supply them with the vitamins and minerals they need, all while keeping an eye on the number of calories they consume. In order to supply the body with the nutrients it requires to fight inflammation, it is essential to include whole grains, fruits, vegetables, lean proteins, and healthy fats in the meals that are consumed on a regular basis. Free radicals can be neutralized and oxidative stress, which has been linked to inflammation, can be reduced by eating foods that are rich in antioxidants, including berries and leafy greens. Foods like these can assist.

Moreover, it is vital to listen to one's body and adapt dietary choices accordingly. Some women may find that certain foods trigger inflammation or digestive discomfort, making it necessary to eliminate or limit those items. Keeping a food diary can be a useful tool for identifying patterns and understanding how specific foods affect individual health.

Additionally, incorporating regular physical activity into daily routines complements the anti-inflammatory diet. Not only does physical activity assist in the maintenance of a healthy weight, but it also improves circulation and strengthens both the muscles and the bones. Walking, swimming, and yoga are examples of low-impact activities that can be especially useful, providing both physical and mental health benefits. In conclusion, when making major alterations to their diet, women over the age of 60 should seek the assistance of qualified dietitians or healthcare specialists during this process. These specialists are able to provide individualized counsel and assistance in the development of a sustainable strategy that is in accordance with the needs of the individual in terms of lifestyle and health. By embracing a holistic approach to nutrition and well-being, women can empower themselves to lead healthier, more vibrant lives while effectively managing inflammation.

Chapter 4: Essential Anti-Inflammatory Foods and Grocery List

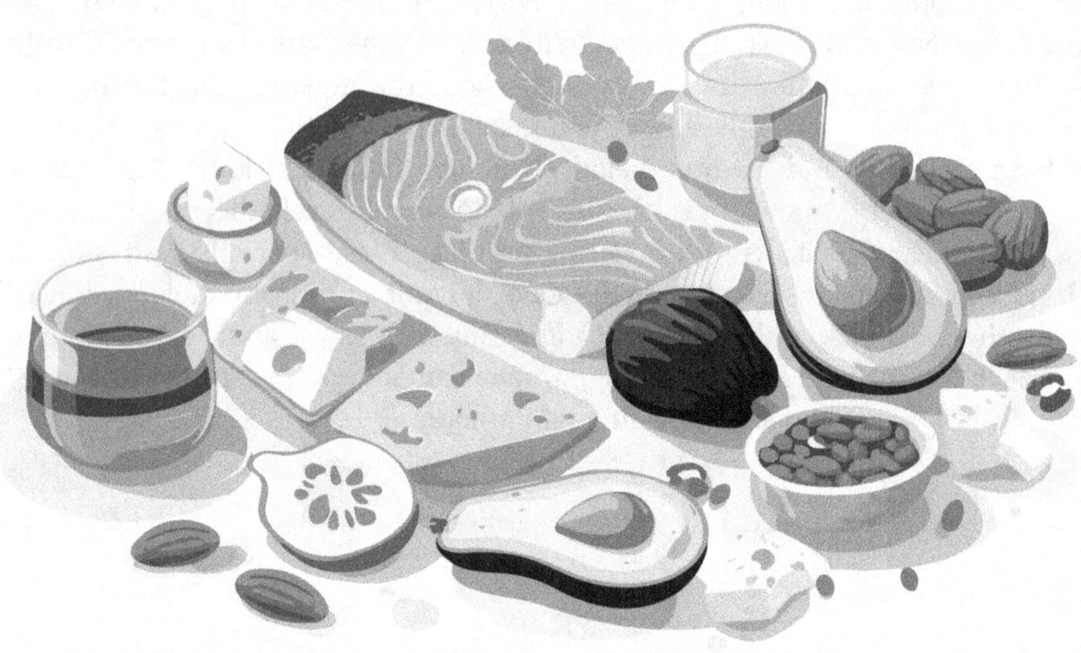

4.1 Whole Grains, Fruits, and Vegetables

Whole grains, fruits, and vegetables are foundational elements of any anti-inflammatory diet, offering a rich array of nutrients that help combat inflammation and support overall health. Whole grains, as opposed to refined grains, which have had their nutrient-rich bran and germ removed, therefore retaining these key components, are a much better option for lowering inflammation than refined grains. Fibre, vitamins, and minerals can be found in abundance in foods like quinoa, brown rice, oats, barley, and whole wheat. These foods are also great sources of fibre. Particularly important is the role that fibre plays in the maintenance of a healthy digestive system and the promotion of a balanced microbiome in the gut, both of which are essential for the regulation of inflammation. Additionally, whole grains include antioxidants and phytonutrients, both of which possess the ability to neutralise potentially harmful free radicals and reduce oxidative stress, which is a significant factor in the development of chronic inflammation.

Fruits and vegetables are equally important in an anti-inflammatory diet due to their high concentration of vitamins, minerals, and **antioxidants**. Brightly colored fruits like berries, oranges, and cherries are packed with compounds such as flavonoids and carotenoids, whose ability to decrease inflammation at the cellular level has been demonstrated. Berries, for instance, include a high concentration of anthocyanins, which are potent antioxidants that promote a reduction in inflammation by preventing the creation of chemicals that can cause inflammation. Fruits that are classified as citrus, such as oranges and grapefruits, contain a significant amount of vitamin C, which is a powerful antioxidant that helps to strengthen the immune system and reduce inflammation.

Vegetables, especially leafy greens like spinach, kale, and collard greens, are some of the most effective anti-inflammatory foods available. These greens are loaded with vitamins A, C, and K, as well as calcium, iron, and magnesium—nutrients that help regulate inflammatory responses in the body. Cruciferous vegetables like broccoli, cauliflower, and Brussels sprouts are also excellent choices, as they contain sulforaphane, a substance that is well-known for its capacity to alleviate inflammation and to give the liver the ability to perform detoxification activities. Furthermore, root vegetables like sweet potatoes and carrots include a high concentration of beta-carotene, which is an antioxidant that causes the body to convert it into vitamin A, which further contributes to the reduction of inflammation. This helps keep stable blood sugar levels and minimise insulin spikes, which can make inflammation worse. Whole grains, fruits, and vegetables also give the benefit of having a **low glycemic index**, which is another benefit of these foods. When individuals make these nutrient-dense, unprocessed meals their top priority, they are able to successfully control inflammation while simultaneously supplying their bodies with the important vitamins and minerals that are required for general health and vigour.

4.2 Omega-3 Rich Foods: Fish, Nuts, and Seeds

Because of their well-documented capacity to decrease inflammation and promote heart health, omega-3 fatty acids are an essential component of any diet that seeks to decrease inflammation. When it comes to the regulation of the body's inflammatory reactions, omega-3 fatty acids, which are a kind of polyunsaturated fat, play a significant role. In contrast to omega-6 fatty acids, which are similarly necessary but can cause inflammation if ingested in excessive amounts, omega-3 fatty acids are needed, omega-3s help to balance the inflammatory process, making them vital for reducing chronic inflammation. Omega-3 fatty acids, in particular eicosapentaenoic acid (EPA) and docosahexaenoic acid (DHA), are found in abundance in fatty fish, like salmon, mackerel, sardines, and trout. These species constitute the greatest sources of omega-3 fatty acids that can be found in the diet. These long-chain omega-3s are especially effective at lowering inflammatory markers in the body and have been associated to a minimized danger of cardiovascular disease, arthritis, and other inflammatory conditions. Regular consumption of fatty fish—at least two servings per week—has been shown to substantially lower levels of C-reactive protein (CRP) and interleukin-6 (IL-6), both of which are key indicators of inflammation. The anti-inflammatory benefits of omega-3s also extend to brain health, according to studies that suggests that these fats may help protect against neuroinflammatory disorders like Alzheimer's disease as well as cognitive decline that is associated with ageing.

In addition to fish, **nuts and seeds** are excellent plant-based sources of omega-3s, particularly alpha-linolenic acid (ALA), a type of omega-3 that the body can convert into EPA and DHA. Walnuts, flaxseeds, chia seeds, and hemp seeds are rich in ALA and offer a convenient and versatile way to increase omega-3 intake. These foods are also high in fiber, protein, and antioxidants, making them beneficial for both reducing inflammation and supporting overall health. For example, flaxseeds contain lignans, a type of phytoestrogen that has been shown to have anti-inflammatory properties, while chia seeds are loaded with fiber and antioxidants that promote gut health and help stabilize blood sugar levels. **Nuts** such as almonds, hazelnuts, and pecans also provide healthy fats, though they are primarily rich in monounsaturated fats rather than omega-3s. While not as concentrated in omega-3s as walnuts or seeds, these nuts still offer anti-inflammatory benefits and are an excellent addition to a balanced diet.

The combination of healthy fats, fiber, and antioxidants in nuts and seeds helps to reduce oxidative stress and inflammation while supporting heart health, brain function, and weight management.

Incorporating both fish and plant-based sources of omega-3s into your diet is an effective strategy for reducing inflammation and promoting long-term health. Whether through grilled salmon, a handful of walnuts, or a sprinkle of flaxseeds on your morning oatmeal, these foods offer a simple yet powerful way to harness the anti-inflammatory power of omega-3s.

4.3 Shopping Tips for Healthy Living

Navigating the grocery store with an anti-inflammatory mindset can make a significant difference in the choices you make, ultimately supporting your overall health. A well-planned shopping strategy is important for maintaining a balanced, anti-inflammatory diet, and this begins with prioritizing whole, unprocessed foods over packaged, refined products. One of the most important tips is to focus on the perimeter of the store, where fresh produce, whole grains, lean proteins, and dairy are typically found. This strategy helps avoid highly processed items often located in the central aisles, which are more likely to contain refined sugars, unhealthy fats, and additives that can trigger inflammation.

When shopping for fruits and vegetables, aim for a **rainbow of colors**. Taking this measure guarantees that you will receive a diverse assortment of vitamins, minerals, and antioxidants, which are key to reducing inflammation. Fresh, seasonal produce is usually the best choice for both flavor and nutrition, but frozen vegetables and fruits can be equally nutritious and convenient, especially for those on a budget or looking for longer-lasting options. Look for frozen produce without added sugars or sauces, as these can detract from their anti-inflammatory benefits.

Another important aspect of healthy grocery shopping is reading labels carefully. Pay close attention to the ingredients list, prioritizing items with simple, whole ingredients. Avoid products with added sugars, artificial preservatives, and trans fats, all of which can promote inflammation. When purchasing packaged foods like whole grain bread, pasta, or cereals, check that they are made with 100% whole grains and contain minimal additives. The fewer ingredients listed on the label, the better the food generally is for your health.

Additionally, it's a good idea to stock up on **healthy fats** such as extra virgin olive oil, avocados, and nuts, which provide anti-inflammatory omega-3 and monounsaturated fats. Choose oils that are cold-pressed and unrefined for maximum nutritional value. Buying in bulk can also be a cost-effective way to stock up on anti-inflammatory staples like whole grains, nuts, seeds, and legumes, allowing you to prepare healthy meals at home without frequent trips to the store.

Planning ahead is another key element to successful shopping for an anti-inflammatory diet. In order to guarantee that you have all of the required components on hand, you should make a weekly meal plan and a grocery list that corresponds to it, helping you avoid impulse purchases of less healthy options. Prepping meals or components of meals ahead of time can make it easier to stick to your diet during busy weeks and slash the temptation to order takeout or rely on processed convenience foods.

Finally, don't forget to include **hydration essentials** in your shopping. Water is crucial for flushing out toxins and supporting your body's anti-inflammatory processes. Herbal teas like ginger, turmeric, and chamomile are excellent additions, as they offer anti-inflammatory benefits while keeping you hydrated throughout the day.

4.4 Supplements That Can Help Reduce Inflammation

In addition to whole foods, certain supplements can play a valuable role in reducing inflammation, particularly for women over 60 who may face specific nutritional challenges. While a well-balanced diet should provide most of the nutrients necessary for fighting inflammation, supplements can offer targeted support where dietary intake might fall short.

Omega-3 supplements, derived from fish oil or algae oil, are among the most effective anti-inflammatory supplements available. If your diet lacks sufficient fatty fish, taking a high-quality omega-3 supplement can help provide the EPA and DHA necessary to lower inflammation and support heart, brain, and joint health. It has been demonstrated that taking omega-3 supplements can lower levels of C-reactive protein (CRP), which is an important indicator of inflammation. This can be especially advantageous for those who suffer from illnesses including arthritis, heart disease, or autoimmune disorders when they take these supplements.

Curcumin, another potent anti-inflammatory substance is turmeric, which contains an active ingredient that is present in turmeric. There has been a significant amount of research conducted on curcumin because of its capacity to inhibit NF-kB, which is a molecule that enters the nuclei of cells and activates genes that are associated with inflammation. However, curcumin is not easily absorbed by the body on its own, so supplements often include piperine, a compound in black pepper, to enhance bioavailability. Taking curcumin supplements can be especially beneficial for reducing joint inflammation, managing arthritis symptoms, and supporting overall inflammatory balance.

Vitamin D is another critical nutrient for inflammation management, particularly for older adults. Low levels of vitamin D have been linked to increased inflammation and a higher risk of chronic conditions such as heart disease and osteoporosis. Since vitamin D is synthesized through sun exposure, many people—especially those who live in northern climates or spend limited time outdoors—may require supplementation to maintain optimal levels. Vitamin D supplements can help regulate the immune system and reduce inflammatory responses, making them an important consideration for women over 60.

Magnesium is another essential mineral that supports anti-inflammatory processes. Many people, particularly older adults, do not get enough magnesium through their diet, which can contribute to increased inflammation. Magnesium supplements help regulate blood sugar levels, support muscle and nerve function, and reduce inflammatory markers. The consumption of foods that are high in magnesium, including nuts, seeds, and leafy greens, is advantageous, but a supplement can help fill any gaps, particularly for individuals with low magnesium levels.

Probiotics are also worth considering, as they support gut health, which is closely linked to inflammation. Regulating the immune system and preventing the development of chemicals that promote inflammation are both benefits of having a healthy microbiome in the stomach. Probiotic supplements can be particularly helpful for individuals who have experienced digestive issues or have taken antibiotics, which can disrupt the balance of gut bacteria.

Lastly, **herbal supplements** like ginger and Boswellia have shown promise in reducing inflammation naturally. Ginger has been shown to have chemicals known as gingerols and shogaols, both of which have anti-inflammatory qualities. Boswellia, commonly known as Indian frankincense, has been utilised for a considerable amount of time in order to alleviate inflammation, particularly in cases of arthritis. Both of these herbal remedies can be taken in supplement form to support the body's natural inflammation-fighting processes.

4.5 Herbal Teas and Natural Remedies

Teas made from herbs and other natural medicines have been utilized for ages in a variety of cultures to assist in the reduction of inflammation and the promotion of general wellness. For women over 60, these natural approaches offer a gentle yet effective way to support the body's anti-inflammatory processes, providing both physical and mental health benefits without the side effects often associated with pharmaceutical interventions.

One of the most well-known anti-inflammatory herbal teas is **turmeric tea**. The spice known as turmeric, which is brilliant yellow in color and is frequently used in Indian cooking, includes a potent component known as curcumins. There is a lot of praise for the anti-inflammatory and antioxidant capabilities that curcumin possesses. Drinking turmeric tea regularly can help reduce chronic inflammation by blocking inflammatory pathways in the body. A little bit of black pepper, which contains piperine, is commonly advised to be added to turmeric tea in order to improve the body's ability to absorb curcumin. Piperine is a component found in black pepper, significantly improves curcumin's bioavailability.

Another excellent herbal tea for inflammation is **ginger tea**. Ginger is associated with the presence of bioactive molecules, like gingerol, which has powerful anti-inflammatory properties. Ginger tea has been shown to be effective in reducing inflammation, particularly in the muscles and joints, making it a popular remedy for individuals with arthritis or other inflammatory conditions. Ginger tea is a wonderful choice for general health since, in addition to its anti-inflammatory effects, it can also help with digestion, promote circulation, and give a relaxing impact on the stomach.

Green tea is another herbal beverage widely praised for its anti-inflammatory benefits. There is a high concentration of polyphenols in green tea, especially epigallocatechin gallate (EGCG), which is a potent antioxidant that has the ability to dampen inflammation and shield cells from the damage that is produced by oxidative stress. Green tea use on a regular basis has been linked to a lower chance of developing chronic diseases such as cardiovascular disease, cancer, and neurological disorders. Its ability to lower inflammatory markers makes green tea a versatile and easily accessible natural remedy for inflammation.

For those looking for a calming, anti-inflammatory tea, **chamomile tea** is an ideal choice. Chamomile has been conventionally used to relieve stress, improve sleep, and reduce inflammation. It contains flavonoids, such as apigenin, which can reduce inflammation and promote relaxation. Chamomile tea can be especially helpful for soothing digestive discomfort and calming the nervous system, making it a great option for women over 60 who may experience stress-related inflammation.

In addition to teas, other **natural remedies** can be integrated into an anti-inflammatory lifestyle. For example, **aloe vera juice** is known for its soothing properties, often used to reduce inflammation both internally and externally. Drinking aloe vera juice can help alleviate inflammation in the digestive tract, particularly for individuals suffering from conditions such as irritable bowel syndrome (IBS) or acid reflux. Aloe vera can be used to the skin outside of the body to alleviate inflammation and speed up the healing process for wounds such as sunburns, cuts, or rashes.

Boswellia, or Indian frankincense, is another natural remedy that has been used for centuries in Ayurvedic medicine for its powerful anti-inflammatory properties. Extracts from the Boswellia tree contain compounds that inhibit the production of inflammatory molecules, consequently, it can be used as a natural treatment for illnesses like asthma and arthritis. Boswellia supplements or teas can be a useful addition to a comprehensive anti-inflammatory plan, especially for women experiencing joint discomfort.

Peppermint tea is yet another herbal option with anti-inflammatory benefits, particularly for digestive health. Peppermint contains menthol, which can relax the muscles of the gastrointestinal tract, easing bloating and digestive discomfort. Its anti-inflammatory effects are especially beneficial for those dealing with conditions like IBS or colitis. Additionally, peppermint tea has a cooling effect, making it refreshing and soothing, particularly during warmer months.

Beyond teas, **essential oils** such as lavender, eucalyptus, and frankincense can be used in aromatherapy or applied topically (when diluted) to reduce inflammation and promote relaxation. **Lavender oil**, for instance, is known for its calming properties and can help alleviate stress-related inflammation. Eucalyptus oil has anti-inflammatory and analgesic properties, making it useful for soothing muscle pain or respiratory inflammation when inhaled through steam or applied in diluted form to the skin.

Lastly, **honey and lemon** are simple yet effective additions to herbal teas. Honey, and more specifically raw or Manuka honey, possesses anti-inflammatory and antibacterial qualities, which makes it a natural way to strengthen the immune system and assist the body's battle against inflammation. The anti-inflammatory properties of teas and remedies can be further enhanced by the addition of lemon, which is abundant in vitamin C and antioxidants. Lemon can also assist to neutralize free radicals while decreasing oxidative stress and inflammation.

Incorporating herbal teas and natural remedies into daily routines is an easy, enjoyable way for women over 60 to harness the power of nature to combat inflammation. These remedies not only provide physical benefits but also offer comfort and relaxation, contributing to a holistic approach to managing inflammation.

Chapter 5: Combining Diet and Exercise for Maximum Results

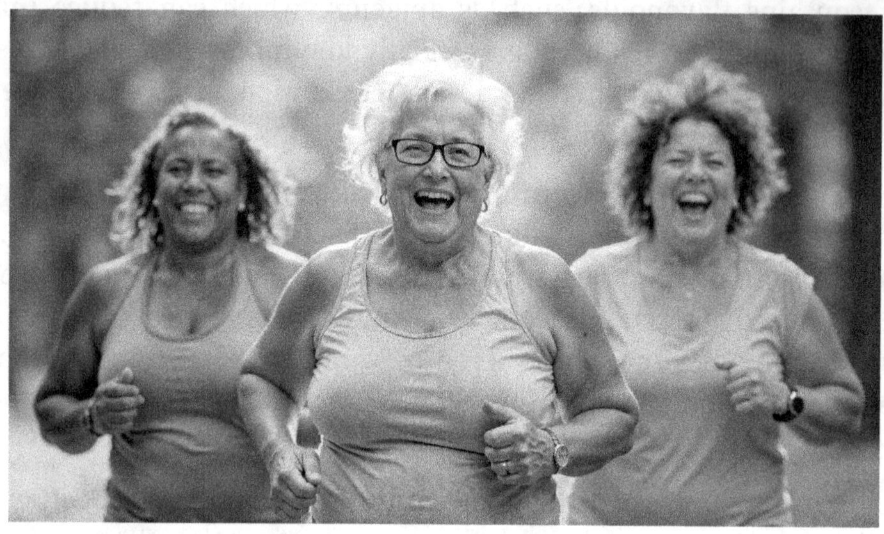

5.1 The Importance of Physical Activity After 60

For women over 60, especially those adopting an anti-inflammatory diet, incorporating physical activity into daily routines can amplify the benefits of a healthy diet, helping to manage inflammation, maintain strength, and promote longevity.

One of the most significant reasons physical activity is crucial after 60 is its ability to **combat inflammation**. Regular exercise has been shown to reduce the production of pro-inflammatory cytokines and increase the release of anti-inflammatory molecules, thereby helping to regulate the body's inflammatory response. For women following an anti-inflammatory diet, adding exercise can create a powerful synergy, where diet and movement work together to reduce chronic inflammation, improve joint health, and support the immune system. Engaging in physical activity also helps mitigate the natural **loss of muscle mass**, or sarcopenia, that occurs with aging. For women over 60, maintaining strong muscles is essential not only for mobility but also for supporting joints, it has the potential to treat illnesses like osteoarthritis, which is a prevalent inflammatory condition that affects people of advanced age. Integrating strength training with a diet that is high in omega-3 fatty acids and antioxidants is an effective anti-inflammatory strategy, and whole foods can further support joint health and reduce pain associated with inflammation. **Bone health** is another critical concern for women over 60. With the decline in estrogen levels post-menopause, bone density tends to decrease, increasing the risk of osteoporosis and fractures. Bone density can be improved by performing weight-bearing exercises such as walking, hiking, or light resistance training. These workouts can help slow the rate of bone loss and stimulate bone development, so boosting bone density overall. These exercises, when combined with an anti-inflammatory diet rich in calcium, vitamin D, and magnesium, has the potential to greatly lower the risk of osteoporosis and to produce bones that are stronger and healthier. After the age of sixty, **heart health** needs to be a key concern as well because the chance of developing heart disease increases with age.

By boosting circulation, lowering blood pressure, and lowering cholesterol levels, regular aerobic activity, like brisk walking, swimming, or cycling, can enhance heart health. This is accomplished by participating in these activities. Furthermore, physical activity helps to regulate blood sugar levels, which is essential for the prevention or management of illnesses such as type 2 diabetes among individuals, which is often associated with inflammation. For women over 60 following an anti-inflammatory diet, cardiovascular exercise can enhance these benefits by improving circulation and reducing the build-up of inflammatory markers in the bloodstream.

Beyond the physical advantages, exercise plays a vital role in **mental well-being**. As women age, they may face emotional challenges such as stress, anxiety, or feelings of isolation, all of which can exacerbate inflammation. Physical activity, particularly low-impact forms such as yoga, tai chi, or stretching exercises, can help reduce stress and promote relaxation. These activities encourage mindfulness and deep breathing, which lowers cortisol levels—a stress hormone that can trigger inflammation when chronically elevated. For women over 60, incorporating mindful movement into daily routines can not only reduce stress but also improve flexibility, balance, and mental clarity, all while supporting an anti-inflammatory lifestyle.

Another key aspect of physical activity is its ability to **enhance metabolism** and promote healthy weight management. As the metabolism naturally slows down with age, it is becoming increasingly difficult to keep a healthy weight, particularly in the abdomen region, where excess fat is often linked to increased inflammation. Exercise helps rev up the metabolism, making it easier to maintain or lose weight, which in turn reduces inflammatory markers such as C-reactive protein (CRP). Coupled with an anti-inflammatory diet that is low in refined sugars and processed foods, exercise can support healthier weight management, reduce visceral fat, and lower the risk of obesity-related inflammation. Flexibility and mobility are equally important components of physical activity for women over 60. Stretching exercises, Pilates, or yoga can help maintain **joint flexibility**, reduce stiffness, and improve posture. This is particularly beneficial for preventing or managing conditions like arthritis, which is marked by chronic inflammation of the joints. By staying mobile and flexible, women over 60 can maintain their independence and reduce the likelihood of injury or pain, which can hinder the pursuit of an active lifestyle. Stretching exercises also promote circulation, allowing nutrients from an anti-inflammatory diet to reach muscles and joints more effectively.

Finally, regular physical activity promotes **longevity and quality of life**. Numerous studies have shown that staying active into older age not only increases lifespan but also improves overall quality of life by maintaining mobility, mental sharpness, and emotional resilience. For women over 60, maintaining a consistent exercise routine can reduce the risk of age-related diseases, improve cognitive function, and foster a sense of vitality. When combined with an anti-inflammatory diet that supports cellular health, these lifestyle changes can help women over 60 enjoy a more active, pain-free life well into their later years.

5.2 30-Day Exercise Plan for Women Over 60

This 30-day exercise plan is designed specifically for women over 60 who are following an anti-inflammatory diet. The exercises focus on improving mobility, strength, flexibility, and cardiovascular health while reducing inflammation. The plan includes a balance of aerobic, strength, and flexibility exercises, along with rest days to allow the body to recover. All exercises are low-impact and suitable for beginners, with the option to modify based on individual fitness levels. Consistency is essential, which is why it is essential to pay attention to your body and make adjustments as required.

WEEK 1: BUILDING A FOUNDATION

> **Day 1: Brisk Walking (20 minutes):** A simple yet effective way to start your exercise routine. Walk at a pace where your heart rate increases, but you can still hold a conversation. Walking helps improve cardiovascular health, circulation, and reduces inflammation.

> **Day 2: Lower Body Strength (20 minutes): Bodyweight Squats (3 sets of 10 reps):** Position your feet so that they are shoulder-width apart. Maintaining a straight back while bending your knees and hips will allow you to lower your body lower. Put some effort into your heels in order to get back to standing. Squats strengthen the legs, glutes, and core, important for maintaining mobility and joint health. **Glute Bridges (3 sets of 10 reps):** Get into a supine position with your knees bent and your feet planted firmly on the ground. Bring your hips up toward the ceiling while contracting your glutes, and then bring them back down to the ground. The glutes and lower back are the muscles that are targeted by this exercise, which helps with hip stability and reduces pain in the lower back.

> **Day 3: Rest Day:** A day of rest is essential for muscle recovery. Focus on hydration and consume anti-inflammatory foods like fruits, vegetables, and omega-3-rich fish.

> **Day 4: Upper Body Strength (20 minutes): Wall Push-ups (3 sets of 10 reps):** With your arms outstretched and your back to the wall, position your hands so that they are at shoulder height on the wall. After bending your elbows and lowering your body toward the wall, you should then push yourself back up. This exercise strengthens the chest, shoulders, and arms while being gentle on the joints. **Bicep Curls with Light Weights (3 sets of 12 reps):** Hold a pair of light dumbbells or water bottles. Curl the weights towards your shoulders, then lower back down. Strengthening the arms is important for daily activities and reducing muscle loss with age.

> **Day 5: Yoga and Stretching (30 minutes): Cat-Cow Stretch:** Make a start on all fours. Make a cat-like arch with your back, then lower your tummy and raise your head to make a cow-like position. This gentle flow increases spinal flexibility and reduces stiffness. **Seated Forward Fold:** Assume a seated position with your legs stretched out in front of you and reach your hands down to your toes. This stretch improves hamstring flexibility and relieves tension in the lower back.

> **Day 6: Rest Day:** Another day for recovery. Use this time to focus on stress reduction techniques, like deep breathing or meditation, which can help lower inflammation.

➤ **Day 7: Gentle Aerobics (20 minutes):** Engage in a low-impact aerobic exercise like **swimming** or **cycling**. These activities boost cardiovascular health without putting too much strain on the joints, making them ideal for women over 60.

WEEK 2: STRENGTHENING AND MOBILITY

➤ **Day 8: Brisk Walking (25 minutes):** Increase the duration slightly to continue building cardiovascular endurance and improve circulation, which helps reduce inflammation.

➤ **Day 9: Lower Body Strength (20 minutes): Step-ups (3 sets of 10 reps per leg):** Using a sturdy step or bench, step up with one leg and then step down. This exercise strengthens the legs and improves balance, essential for joint stability and fall prevention. **Seated Leg Lifts (3 sets of 10 reps per leg):** Place both of your feet firmly on the ground and sit down on a chair. Put one leg out in a straight position, hold for a second, and then lower. This exercise targets the quadriceps and improves knee joint stability.

➤ **Day 10: Rest Day**

➤ **Day 11: Core Strength (20 minutes): Seated Russian Twists (3 sets of 12 reps):** When you are seated on the floor, bend your knees and place your feet flat. Perform a side-to-side twist with your torso while holding a weight (or no weight at all). This exercise strengthens the obliques and improves core stability. **Plank (3 sets of 15-30 seconds):** Begin by placing your hands on your forearms and assuming a push-up position. Maintain a straight line with your body while working your core muscles. Planks improve core strength, which supports posture and reduces back pain.

➤ **Day 12: Yoga for Flexibility (30 minutes): Warrior I and II Poses:** These standing poses strengthen the legs while stretching the chest, shoulders, and groin. Yoga also enhances mental clarity and reduces stress-related inflammation.

➤ **Day 13: Rest Day**

➤ **Day 14: Low-Impact Cardio (30 minutes):** Engage in a gentle cardio session like **dancing** or **water aerobics**. These activities provide full-body movement, improving cardiovascular endurance and overall flexibility.

WEEK 3: INCREASING INTENSITY

➤ **Day 15: Brisk Walking (30 minutes):** Continue building cardiovascular endurance by increasing your walking time.

➤ **Day 16: Total Body Strength (30 minutes):** Combine **lower body exercises** (squats, step-ups) and **upper body exercises** (wall push-ups, bicep curls) into a full-body workout.

➤ **Day 17: Rest Day**

➤ **Day 18: Core and Balance (20 minutes): Single-Leg Balance (3 sets of 15 seconds per leg):** Stand on one leg and hold the position. This exercise improves balance and stability, important for preventing falls as we age. **Dead Bug (3 sets of 10 reps per side):** Lie down on your back with your knees bent at a 90-degree angle and your arms extended above your head toward the sky. The next step is to return to the starting posture after lowering one arm and the opposing leg towards the floor first. This core exercise improves coordination and abdominal strength.

➤ **Day 19: Stretching and Relaxation (30 minutes): Child's Pose and Pigeon Pose:** These stretches target the hips and lower back, promoting flexibility and reducing inflammation.

➤ **Day 20: Rest Day**

➤ **Day 21: Aerobic Exercise (30 minutes):** Choose a favorite aerobic activity, such as **light hiking**, to keep your body moving while enjoying nature and reducing stress.

WEEK 4: MAINTAINING AND PROGRESSING

➤ **Day 22: Brisk Walking (30 minutes)**

➤ **Day 23: Strength Training (20 minutes):** Continue with a full-body strength session, increasing the number of repetitions or adding light weights if comfortable.

➤ **Day 24: Rest Day**

➤ **Day 25: Yoga for Strength and Flexibility (30 minutes):** Incorporate a variety of poses that stretch and strengthen the entire body, focusing on breathing to reduce stress.

➤ **Day 26: Rest Day**

➤ **Day 27: Low-Impact Cardio (30 minutes)**

➤ **Day 28: Total Body Strength (30 minutes)**

➤ **Day 29: Rest Day**

➤ **Day 30: Full-Body Stretching and Reflection (30 minutes):** Spend time doing gentle stretches to release tension, improve flexibility, and reflect on the progress made over the last 30 days.

5.3 Lifestyle Changes to Support an Anti-Inflammatory Diet

Adopting an anti-inflammatory diet requires more than just adjusting what's on your plate; it often involves making significant lifestyle changes to support and maintain long-term health benefits. For women over 60, these changes are particularly important, as aging introduces new challenges like hormonal shifts, reduced metabolism, and an increased susceptibility to chronic inflammation. One essential lifestyle change is to prioritize stress management. Chronic stress is one of the most potent triggers of inflammation in the body. Women over 60 might face various stressors, from adjusting to retirement to managing health concerns or family dynamics. In order to avoid chronic inflammation that can develop to illnesses such as heart disease, arthritis, and diabetes, it is essential to discover efficient methods of stress management. Mindfulness meditation and exercises that focus on deep breathing are examples of such practices, and even light yoga or tai chi can significantly reduce cortisol levels, the hormone responsible for stress, thereby lowering inflammatory responses. Another key change is improving sleep habits. As we age, getting sufficient, restful sleep becomes more challenging due to changes in sleep patterns and hormone levels. Poor sleep quality is closely linked to increased inflammation. Developing a consistent pattern of sleep, which includes going to bed and waking up at the same time every day, limiting coffee and heavy meals in the hours leading up to bedtime, and creating a sleep environment that is conducive to relaxation and rest—can help ensure deeper, restorative sleep, which is vital for immune system function and cellular repair. Additionally, adopting a more active lifestyle is crucial. Reducing prolonged periods of sedentary behavior is necessary for managing inflammation. This could mean simple adjustments like standing up and moving around for a few minutes every hour, integrating light exercises throughout the day, or opting for activities like gardening, which keep the body active and engaged without overwhelming the joints.

Sleep, Stress Management, and Mental Well-being

Sleep, stress management, and mental well-being are three interconnected pillars that profoundly affect inflammation levels, particularly for women over 60. Post-menopausal changes often lead to sleep disturbances, such as difficulty falling or staying asleep, which can have a cascading effect on overall health. Insufficient sleep has been shown to increase the production of pro-inflammatory cytokines, proteins that signal inflammation in the body. As women age, the body's ability to regulate these inflammatory responses declines, making restful sleep even more critical. To promote better sleep, it's essential to establish good sleep hygiene. This includes creating a relaxing bedtime routine, limiting screen time an hour before sleep, and ensuring the bedroom is a calm, dark, and quiet environment. The inclusion of herbal teas, like chamomile or valerian root, can naturally support relaxation and improve sleep quality without the need for medication.

Stress is another significant factor that can exacerbate inflammation. For women in their 60s, dealing with life transitions—such as retirement, changes in social roles, or health challenges—can create emotional and mental strain. Prolonged stress elevates cortisol levels, which over time contributes to chronic inflammation. Managing stress is not just about reducing discomfort in the moment but about preventing long-term damage to the body.

In order to effectively reduce stress, it is essential to implement stress-reduction strategies, like indulging in activities that bring joy and relaxation or practicing mindfulness meditation. Additionally, regular exercise has been proven to lower stress and anxiety levels by increasing the release of endorphins, the body's natural mood elevators. Whether it's through walking in nature, participating in group classes, or practicing yoga, movement serves as both a physical and emotional release, promoting mental well-being.

Mental well-being is deeply tied to how the body handles inflammation. Women over 60 may experience shifts in mental health due to hormonal changes, retirement, or changing family dynamics, which can lead to feelings of isolation or depression. Staying mentally active—whether through social engagement, learning new skills, or pursuing creative outlets—is just as important as staying physically active. By nurturing mental and emotional health, women can maintain a positive outlook, which in turn helps regulate inflammatory processes in the body.

The Role of Hydration and Detoxification

Hydration plays a critical role in maintaining health, especially for women over 60 who are on an anti-inflammatory diet. As the body ages, the sensation of thirst becomes less acute, meaning older adults may not feel the need to drink water as often as younger individuals. Dehydration can exacerbate inflammation and contribute to issues such as joint pain, dry skin, and kidney dysfunction. Staying well-hydrated helps flush toxins from the body, aids digestion, and supports overall cellular health, making it a vital part of an anti-inflammatory lifestyle. Drinking adequate amounts of water also aids in detoxification, a natural process where the body eliminates waste and toxins. While the liver, kidneys, and lymphatic system are the primary organs responsible for detoxifying the body, staying hydrated ensures that these organs function efficiently. Women over 60 should aim to drink at least 8-10 glasses of water per day, adjusting based on activity levels or climate. Herbal teas, especially those known for their anti-inflammatory properties like green tea, turmeric tea, or ginger tea, can also contribute to hydration while offering additional benefits.

In addition to hydration, incorporating detoxifying foods into the diet can further enhance the body's natural ability to reduce inflammation. Foods rich in antioxidants, such as berries, leafy greens, and cruciferous vegetables, support liver function and neutralize free radicals, which can cause cellular damage and inflammation. Omega-3-rich foods, like fatty fish and flaxseeds, also promote detoxification by reducing oxidative stress in the body.

Physical activity complements this detoxification process by increasing circulation, promoting sweat, and aiding lymphatic drainage. Exercise, combined with proper hydration, creates an optimal environment for the body to eliminate toxins and regulate inflammatory responses. By prioritizing both hydration and detoxification, women over 60 can enhance the benefits of their anti-inflammatory diet, supporting overall health and well-being.

Chapter 6: Anti-Inflammatory Breakfast Recipes

1. Turmeric Oatmeal with Blueberries and Almonds

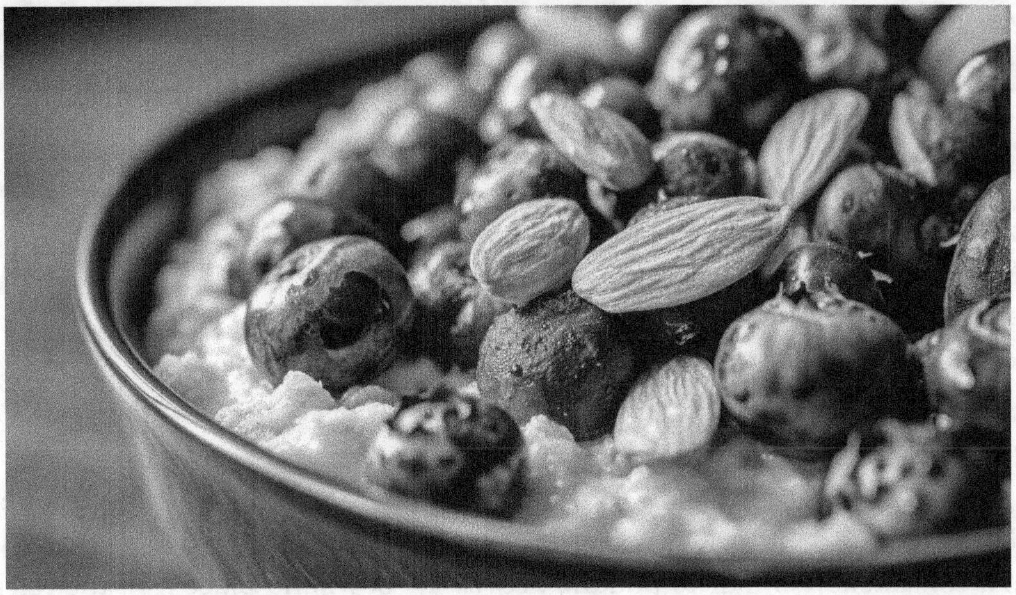

This anti-inflammatory oatmeal is perfect for women over 60. Turmeric's potent anti-inflammatory properties, combined with fiber-rich oats, antioxidant-packed blueberries, and heart-healthy almonds, make this breakfast a great choice for reducing joint pain, improving digestion, and boosting overall health.

(Ready in: 10 minutes | Cook Duration: 5mins | Persons: 2)

Necessary Items:

- Rolled oats: 1 cup
- Almond milk (or other non-dairy milk): 2 cups
- Ground turmeric: 1/2 tsp
- Cinnamon: 1/4 tsp
- Fresh or frozen blueberries: 1/2 cup
- Almonds (sliced or severed): 2 tbsps
- Honey or maple syrup (optional, as required): 1 tbsp
- Ground black pepper: a pinch (to enhance turmeric absorption)

How to Prepare. Put the oats, almond milk, turmeric, cinnamon, and black pepper into a pot and mix them together evenly. While tossing the mixture on occasions continue cooking the oats over middling temp. for 5 minutes, or until they have become mushy and have absorbed the liquid. After it has finished cooking, take it off the heat and allow it settle for a minute. Divide the oatmeal into bowls, and top with fresh or frozen blueberries, almonds, and honey or maple syrup if desired. Present warm and enjoy.

Nutritional Info (per serving): Calories: 250 kcal, Protein: 7g, Carbohydrates: 38g, Fat: 9g, Fiber: 6g, Sugars: 11g, Sodium: 80mg

2. Chia Seed Pudding with Mixed Berries

This simple chia seed pudding is loaded with omega-3s, fiber, and antioxidants, in women over the age of sixty, all of these are vital for lowering inflammation, encouraging good digestion, and supporting the health of cardiovascular systems. The combination of berries provides a boost of vitamin C and adds a touch of sweetness that comes from nature.

(Ready in: 10 minutes - plus overnight chilling | Cook Duration: 25 minutes | Persons: 2)

Necessary Items:

- Chia seeds: 1/4 cup
- Unsweetened almond milk (or other non-dairy milk): 1 cup
- Vanilla extract: 1/2 tsp
- Mixed berries (fresh or frozen): 1/2 cup
- Honey or maple syrup (optional, as required): 1 tbsp
- Almonds or walnuts (optional, for topping): 2 tbsps

How to Prepare: The chia seeds, almond milk, and vanilla essence should be mixed collectively in a bowl using a whisk. To ensure that there are no chia seed lumps, give the mixture a thorough stir to integrate it. In order to give the chia seeds the opportunity to expand and develop a consistency similar to pudding, cover the bowl and place it in the refrigerator for almost 4 hours or overnight. When it is ready, give the pudding another stir to check that it is consistent. Divide into bowls and top with mixed berries and nuts if desired. As an additional sweetener, you may also drizzle honey or maple syrup over the dish. Present chilled and enjoy!

Nutritional Info: Calories: 190 kcal, Protein: 5g, Carbohydrates: 24g, Fat: 9g, Fiber: 11g, Sugars: 8g, Sodium: 40mg

3. Avocado Toast with Smoked Salmon and Microgreens

Avocado toast has become a breakfast staple, and for good reason. Packed with healthy fats from the avocado, omega-3s from smoked salmon, and nutrient-dense microgreens, this dish helps reduce inflammation, supports heart health, and promotes joint flexibility. I

(Ready in: 15 minutes | Serves: 2)

Ingredients:

- Whole-grain or gluten-free bread: 2 pieces
- Ripe avocado: 1
- Smoked salmon: 2 oz.
- Lemon juice: 1 tsp
- Olive oil: 1 tsp
- Microgreens or arugula: 1/4 cup
- Salt and pepper: as required
- Red pepper flakes (optional): a pinch

Instructions: The pieces of whole-grain bread should be toasted until they are golden brown and crunchy. While the bread is being toasted, mash the avocado in a bowl and combine it with the lemon juice, olive oil, salt, and pepper according to your taste. The mashed avocado mixture should be spread out evenly over the bread that has been toasted.

Layer the smoked salmon on top of the avocado. Garnish with fresh microgreens and a sprinkle of red pepper flakes if you like a bit of spice.

Nutritional Info: Calories: 280 kcal, Protein: 12g, Carbohydrates: 20g, Fat: 19g, Fiber: 7g, Sugars: 2g, Sodium: 350mg

4. Quinoa Breakfast Bowl with Walnuts and Pomegranate Seeds

This quinoa breakfast bowl is rich in plant-based protein and fiber, making it an ideal option for women over 60 following an anti-inflammatory diet. Quinoa helps stabilize blood sugar, while walnuts provide omega-3 fatty acids, and pomegranate seeds offer antioxidants that fight inflammation and support overall health.

(Ready in: 15 minutes | Cook Duration: 15 minutes | Persons: 2)

Necessary Items:

- Quinoa (uncooked): 1/2 cup
- Water: 1 cup
- Walnuts (severed): 2 tbsps
- Pomegranate seeds: 1/4 cup
- Almond milk (or other non-dairy milk): 1/4 cup
- Honey or maple syrup (optional, as required): 1 tbsp
- Cinnamon: 1/4 tsp
- Ground flaxseeds (optional): 1 tbsp

How to Prepare: To eliminate any traces of bitterness, the quinoa should be washed in cold water. To prepare the quinoa, blend it with the water in a small saucepan. Raise the mixture to a boil, and then decrease the temp. to a simmer. The quinoa should be cooked for 12 to 15 minutes, or until the water has been absorbed and it has become fluffy. Once it is cooked, take it from the temp. and let it cool down a little bit. After the quinoa has been cooked, blend it with the almond milk and cinnamon in a bowl and toss it thoroughly. Top the quinoa with severed walnuts, pomegranate seeds, and ground flaxseeds if desired. Additional sweetness can be achieved by drizzling honey or maple syrup over the top. Keep warm and savor the dish.

Nutritional Info: Calories: 320 kcal, Protein: 9g, Carbohydrates: 42g, Fat: 14g, Fiber: 6g, Sugars: 10g, Sodium: 10mg

5. Greek Yogurt with Flaxseeds and Honey

Greek yogurt is an excellent source of protein and probiotics, supporting gut health and aiding digestion for women over 60. Flaxseeds provide omega-3 fatty acids and fiber, which reduce inflammation and support heart health. The addition of honey offers a natural sweetness, making this a quick and nourishing breakfast.

(Ready in: 5 minutes | Persons: 2)

Necessary Items:

- Plain Greek yogurt (unsweetened): 1 cup
- Flaxseeds (ground): 1 tbsp
- Honey: 1 tbsp
- Fresh berries (optional): 1/2 cup

- Walnuts (optional, for topping): 2 tbsps

How to Prepare: Greek yogurt should be spooned into a bowl, and then powdered flaxseeds should be stirred in. Honey is drizzled over the yogurt, and then the mixture is stirred to blend. Top with fresh berries and walnuts if desired, for added antioxidants and healthy fats.

Nutritional Info: Calories: 200 kcal, Protein: 14g, Carbohydrates: 22g, Fat: 7g, Fiber: 3g, Sugars: 15g, Sodium: 65mg

---

6. Buckwheat Pancakes with Fresh Raspberries

Buckwheat is a naturally gluten-free grain that is high in fiber and antioxidants, making these pancakes a healthy, anti-inflammatory breakfast choice for women over 60. The incorporation of fresh raspberries offers a substantial quantity of vitamin C and fiber, both of which contribute to the function of the immune system and the health of the digestive system.

(Ready in: 10 mins | SCook Duration: 15 minutes | Persons: 2)

Ingredients:

- Buckwheat flour: 1/2 cup
- Egg: 1 large
- Almond milk (or any non-dairy milk): 1/2 cup
- Baking powder: 1/2 tsp
- Vanilla extract: 1/2 tsp
- Cinnamon: 1/4 tsp
- Coconut oil (for cooking): 1 tbsp
- Fresh raspberries: 1/2 cup
- Maple syrup (optional, for presenting): 2 tbsps

Instructions: A bowl should be used to combine the buckwheat flour, baking powder, and cinnamon by whisking them together. The egg should be beaten in a separate bowl, and then it should be combined with almond milk and vanilla extract. Mix the dry components with the wet ones in a slow and steady manner until they are completely incorporated. Coconut oil should be used to mildly coat a non-stick pan before it is heated from medium to high. It is possible to make pancakes by pouring little amounts of batter into the pan. 2 to 3 minutes on all sides, or until bubbles appear on the surface, should be spent cooking. Top with fresh raspberries and drizzle with maple syrup if desired. Present warm.

Nutritional Info: Calories: 290 kcal, Protein: 8g, Carbohydrates: 36g, Fat: 12g, Fiber: 5g, Sugars: 10g, Sodium: 160mg

---

7. Anti-Inflammatory Green Smoothie with Kale and Pineapple

This vibrant green smoothie is packed with kale, a nutrient-dense leafy green, and pineapple, which contains bromelain, a natural anti-inflammatory enzyme. The combination of these ingredients makes it an excellent choice for reducing inflammation and promoting overall health, particularly for women over 60.

(Ready in: 5 minutes | Persons: 2)

Necessary Items:

- Fresh kale (stems taken out): 1 cup
- Fresh pineapple (cubed): 1/2 cup
- Banana: 1 small
- Almond milk (or other non-dairy milk): 1 cup
- Ground ginger: 1/2 tsp
- Chia seeds: 1 tbsp
- Ice cubes (optional): 1/2 cup

How to Prepare: Kale, pineapple, banana, almond milk, ground ginger, and chia seeds should all be placed in a mixer. Blend until smooth. Puree till it is silky smooth and creamy. Include ice cubes and blend once more until everything is completely incorporated if you want the consistency to be thicker. Prepare the smoothie by pouring it into glasses and serving it right away.

Nutritional Info: Calories: 180 kcal, Protein: 4g, Carbohydrates: 32g, Fat: 4g, Fiber: 6g, Sugars: 18g, Sodium: 55mg

8. Cinnamon-Spiced Apple and Almond Porridge

This warm and comforting porridge is an ideal anti-inflammatory breakfast, rich in fiber from oats and apples. Cinnamon, in addition to enhancing the flavor, also contributes to the regulation of blood sugar levels and the reduction of inflammation, making this recipe perfect for women over 60 looking to improve their health through diet.

(Ready in: 10 minutes | Cook Duration: 10 min | Persons: 2)

Necessary Items:

- Rolled oats: 1/2 cup
- Almond milk (or other non-dairy milk): 1 cup
- Apple (severed): 1 small
- Ground cinnamon: 1/2 tsp
- Almond butter: 1 tbsp
- Flaxseeds (ground): 1 tbsp
- Honey or maple syrup (optional, as required): 1 tbsp

How to Prepare: Put the rolled oats and the almond milk into a small saucepan and mix them together. Once it reaches a boil, decrease the temp. and let it simmer for approximately 5 minutes while mixing it irregularly. After adding the severed apple and cinnamon, continue to cook the mixture for approximately an additional 5 minutes, or until the oats have become mushy and the apple has become tender. Mix in the flaxseeds and almond butter until they are completely incorporated into the mixture. If you want to add some sweetness, you can drizzle honey or maple syrup over the top. Present warm.

Nutritional Info: Calories: 280 kcal, Protein: 7g, Carbohydrates: 45g, Fat: 9g, Fiber: 7g, Sugars: 16g, Sodium: 70mg

9. Coconut Yogurt Parfait with Chia and Hemp Seeds

This coconut yogurt parfait is a delicious, dairy-free option packed with anti-inflammatory benefits. The chia and hemp seeds provide omega-3 fatty acids, which help fight inflammation, while the coconut yogurt offers a light, creamy texture. Perfect for women over 60 looking for a nutritious, easy-to-prepare breakfast that supports joint and heart health.

(Ready in: 5 minutes | Cook Duration: None | Persons: 2)

Necessary Items:

- Coconut yogurt (unsweetened): 1 cup
- Chia seeds: 1 tbsp
- Hemp seeds: 1 tbsp
- Fresh mixed berries: 1/2 cup
- Unsweetened shredded coconut: 2 tbsps
- Honey or maple syrup (optional, as required): 1 tbsp

How to Prepare: The coconut yogurt, chia seeds, and hemp seeds should be layered in a bowl or glass separating them. A layer of fresh mixed berries should be added. If you so wish, you can choose to drizzle honey or maple syrup over the top and sprinkle with shredded coconut.

Nutritional Info: Calories: 240 kcal, Protein: 7g, Carbohydrates: 18g, Fat: 15g, Fiber: 6g, Sugars: 10g, Sodium: 20mg

10. Flaxseed and Blueberry Smoothie Bowl

This flaxseed and blueberry smoothie bowl is an antioxidant-rich breakfast that is both filling and nutritious. The flaxseeds provide fiber and omega-3s, while the blueberries are packed with antioxidants, making this bowl an excellent choice for women over 60 to support their cognitive and heart health while reducing inflammation.

(Ready in: 5 minutes | Cook Duration: None | Persons: 2)

Ingredients:

- Frozen blueberries: 1 cup
- Banana: 1 small
- Almond milk (or other non-dairy milk): 1/2 cup
- Ground flaxseeds: 1 tbsp
- Almond butter: 1 tbsp
- Granola (optional, for topping): 1/4 cup
- Fresh berries (for topping): 1/4 cup
- Chia seeds (optional, for topping): 1 tsp

Instructions: Almond butter, ground flaxseeds, frozen blueberries, and banana should be blended together in a blender. Almond milk should also be used. Puree till it is silky smooth and creamy. The smoothie should be poured into a bowl. If you so wish, you may finish it off with granola, fresh berries, and chia seeds.

Nutritional Info: Calories: 320 kcal, Protein: 7g, Carbohydrates: 48g, Fat: 12g, Fiber: 10g, Sugars: 22g, Sodium: 50mg

11. Almond Butter and Banana Rice Cakes

These almond butter and banana rice cakes make for a quick, anti-inflammatory breakfast or snack. Almond butter is rich in healthy fats and vitamin E, which helps combat inflammation, while bananas offer potassium to support muscle function.

(Ready in: 5 minutes | Cook Duration: None | Persons: 2)

Ingredients:

- Whole grain rice cakes: 2
- Almond butter (unsweetened): 2 tbsps
- Ripe banana: 1, sliced
- Cinnamon: 1/4 tsp
- Chia seeds (optional): 1 tsp

Instructions: Spread 1 tbsp of almond butter over each rice cake. Top with banana pieces and a sprinkle of cinnamon. For added crunch and nutrients, sprinkle with chia seeds if desired.

Nutritional Info: Calories: 220 kcal, Protein: 6g, Carbohydrates: 27g, Fat: 11g, Fiber: 5g, Sugars: 8g, Sodium: 60mg

12. Herb Omelet with Avocado and Arugula

This herb omelet is a fantastic protein-rich meal that's both anti-inflammatory and satisfying. Fresh herbs like parsley and chives provide antioxidants, while the avocado and arugula add healthy fats and fiber. For women over 60, this omelet supports muscle health and helps keep inflammation in check.

(Ready in: 10 minutes | Cook Duration: 5 minutes | Persons: 2)

Necessary Items:

- Eggs: 4
- Fresh parsley (severed): 1 tbsp
- Fresh chives (severed): 1 tbsp
- Olive oil: 1 tsp
- Ripe avocado: 1/2, sliced
- Arugula: 1 cup
- Salt and pepper as required

How to Prepare: The eggs should be whisked in a bowl, and then the parsley, chives, salt, and pepper should be stirred in. In a skillet that does not stick, bring the olive oil to a middling temp. The egg mixture should be poured into the pan, and it should be cooked until the edges start to solidify. The edges should be lifted gently with a spatula, and the pan should be tilted so that the raw egg may flow to the edges. Once fully cooked, fold the omelet in half and remove from the pan. Present topped with sliced avocado and a side of fresh arugula for added fiber and nutrients.

Nutritional Info: Calories: 290 kcal, Protein: 14g, Carbohydrates: 7g, Fat: 24g, Fiber: 5g, Sugars: 1g, Sodium: 160mg

13. Pumpkin and Ginger Smoothie

This pumpkin and ginger smoothie is an autumn-inspired, anti-inflammatory treat. Pumpkin is rich in beta-carotene, which helps reduce inflammation and support eye health, while ginger is known for its potent anti-inflammatory properties. This is a nourishing and flavorful option for women over 60 looking to boost their immune system and manage inflammation.

(Ready in: 5 minutes | Cook Duration: None | Persons: 2)

Necessary Items:

- Pumpkin puree (unsweetened): 1/2 cup
- Banana: 1 small, frozen
- Almond milk (or other non-dairy milk): 1 cup
- Ground ginger: 1/2 tsp
- Cinnamon: 1/4 tsp
- Vanilla extract: 1/2 tsp
- Honey or maple syrup (optional): 1 tbsp
- Ice cubes (optional): 1/2 cup

How to Prepare: Put the pumpkin puree, frozen banana, almond milk, ginger, cinnamon, vanilla essence, and ice cubes into a mixer. Blend until smooth. Puree till it is silky smooth and creamy. If you want your smoothie to be sweeter, taste it and perhaps include some honey or maple syrup. Pour into glasses and serve immediately

Nutritional Info: Calories: 180 kcal, Protein: 3g, Carbohydrates: 36g, Fat: 4g, Fiber: 5g, Sugars: 19g, Sodium: 85mg

14. Zucchini and Carrot Breakfast Fritters

These zucchini and carrot fritters are a savory, vegetable-packed breakfast option that provides fiber, vitamins, and anti-inflammatory benefits. Zucchini and carrots are both rich in antioxidants, while the fritters offer a satisfying crunch without inflammatory oils.

(Ready in: 20 minutes | Cook Duration: 10 minutes | Persons: 2)

Necessary Items:

- Zucchini (grated): 1 medium
- Carrots (grated): 1 large
- Eggs: 2
- Almond flour: 1/4 cup
- Ground flaxseeds: 1 tbsp
- Garlic powder: 1/2 tsp
- Salt and pepper as required
- Olive oil: 2 tsps

How to Prepare: Grate the zucchini and carrots, then squeeze out excess moisture using a clean kitchen towel. Grated veggies, eggs, almond flour, ground flaxseeds, garlic powder, salt, and pepper should be mixed together in a bowl before being included to the vegetables. Olive oil should be heated in a skillet that does not stick at middling temp. The mixture should be dropped into the skillet in spoonfuls, and then a spatula should be used to gradually flatten it. Approximately 3 to 4 minutes on all sides, until the food is golden brown and crispy. Present warm.

Nutritional Info: Calories: 250 kcal, Protein: 10g, Carbohydrates: 12g, Fat: 18g, Fiber: 5g, Sugars: 5g, Sodium: 200mg

15. Coconut Flour Waffles with Mixed Berries

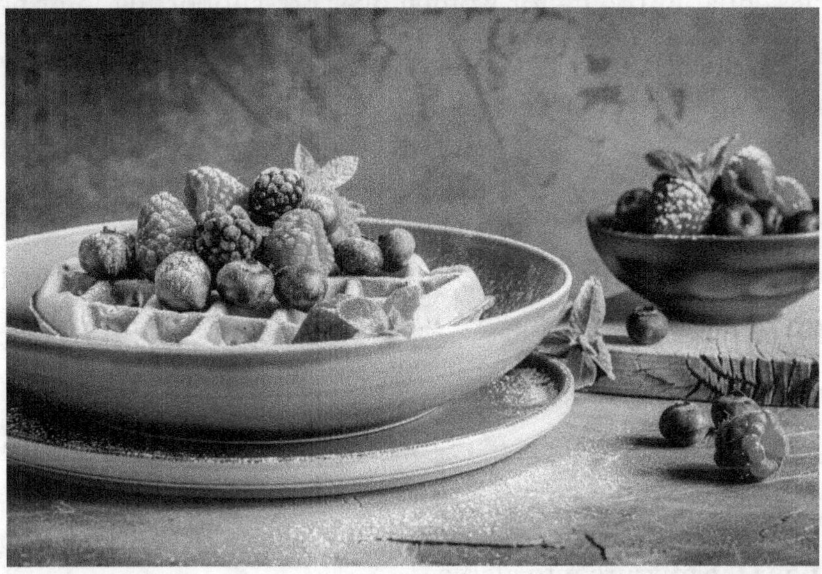

These coconut flour waffles are a gluten-free, low-carb breakfast option that's light yet filling. Coconut flour is a great anti-inflammatory alternative to traditional flours, and when topped with antioxidant-rich mixed berries, this dish becomes a perfect choice for women over 60 who want a nourishing, tasty breakfast.

(Ready in: 15 minutes | Cook Duration: 10 minutes | Persons: 2)

Necessary Items:

- Coconut flour: 1/4 cup
- Eggs: 3
- Almond milk (or other non-dairy milk): 1/4 cup
- Coconut oil (melted): 2 tbsps
- Baking powder: 1/2 tsp
- Vanilla extract: 1/2 tsp
- Fresh mixed berries: 1/2 cup
- Maple syrup (optional): 2 tbsps

How to Prepare: Preheat your waffle iron. Put the eggs, almond milk, melted coconut oil, and vanilla extract into a bowl and whisk them together until they are combined. Using a stirring motion, gradually include the coconut flour and baking powder until a smooth mixture is formed. After the waffle iron has been warmed up, pour the batter into it and fry it in accordance with the directions provided by the manufacturer until it is golden brown and crisp. Depending on your preferences, you can present the waffles with a drizzle of maple syrup and fresh mixed berries on top.

Nutritional Info: Calories: 310 kcal, Protein: 10g, Carbohydrates: 20g, Fat: 22g, Fiber: 6g, Sugars: 10g, Sodium: 150mg

16. Matcha Smoothie with Spinach and Coconut Milk

This matcha smoothie is an energizing breakfast option packed with anti-inflammatory ingredients. Matcha provides antioxidants and a gentle caffeine boost, while spinach and coconut milk offer essential nutrients for women over 60, supporting joint health and reducing inflammation.

(Ready in: 5 minutes | Cook Duration: None | Persons: 2)

Ingredients:

- Matcha powder: 1 tsp
- Fresh spinach: 1 cup
- Coconut milk (unsweetened): 1 cup
- Banana: 1 small, frozen
- Chia seeds: 1 tbsp
- Honey or maple syrup (optional): 1 tbsp
- Ice cubes (optional): 1/2 cup

Instructions: In a mixer, blend the matcha powder, spinach, coconut milk, frozen banana, chia seeds, and ice cubes. Blend until smooth. Puree till it is silky smooth and creamy. It is recommended to taste the mixture and include honey or maple syrup if you want it to be sweeter. To relish, pour the mixture into glasses.

Nutritional Info: Calories: 180 kcal, Protein: 3g, Carbohydrates: 29g, Fat: 8g, Fiber: 5g, Sugars: 12g, Sodium: 55mg

17. Poached Eggs with Avocado and Sautéed Greens

This savory breakfast is rich in anti-inflammatory fats and essential nutrients. Poached eggs provide high-quality protein, while avocado and sautéed greens like spinach or kale offer heart-healthy fats and antioxidants, making it a perfect meal for women over 60 looking to manage inflammation and maintain muscle health.

(Ready in: 15 minutes | Cook Duration: 10 minutes | Persons: 2)

Necessary Items:

- Eggs: 4
- Avocado: 1, sliced
- Spinach or kale: 2 cups
- Olive oil: 1 tbsp
- Garlic (crushed): 1 piece
- Lemon juice: 1 tsp
- Salt and pepper as required

How to Prepare: Poach the eggs by simmering water in a pan and gently dropping each egg in, after around 4 to 5 minutes of cooking, the whites should be firm while the yolks should still be liquid. Prepare the olive oil in a distinct skillet by heating it at middling temp. Sauté the garlic until it achieves a fragrant state. To wilt the spinach or kale, include it to the pan and sauté it for 3 to 4 minutes. Lemon juice should be drizzled on top, and then salt and pepper ought to be included. Present the poached eggs over the sautéed greens, topped with avocado pieces.

Nutritional Info: Calories: 320 kcal, Protein: 14g, Carbohydrates: 12g, Fat: 25g, Fiber: 7g, Sugars: 1g, Sodium: 150mg

18. Cinnamon Quinoa with Almond Milk and Cherries

(Ready in: 20 minutes | Cook Duration: 15 minutes | Persons: 2)

Necessary Items:

- Quinoa: 1/2 cup
- Almond milk (unsweetened): 1 cup
- Fresh or frozen cherries: 1/2 cup
- Cinnamon: 1/2 tsp
- Almond butter: 1 tbsp
- Honey or maple syrup (optional): 1 tbsp

How to Prepare: After giving the quinoa a quick rinse in cold water, place it in a pot along with some almond milk. Bring to a boil, then down the temp. to a simmer and continue cooking for around 15 minutes, or until the quinoa is tender and the liquid has been absorbed. Stir in the cinnamon and almond butter. Present in bowls, topping with cherries and, if preferred, a drizzle of honey or maple syrup on top of the dessert.

Nutritional Info: Calories: 290 kcal, Protein: 8g, Carbohydrates: 39g, Fat: 12g, Fiber: 5g, Sugars: 10g, Sodium: 75mg

19. Almond Flour Muffins with Turmeric and Ginger

These almond flour muffins are a perfect anti-inflammatory snack or breakfast, featuring the powerful combination of turmeric and ginger. Almond flour provides healthy fats and protein, supporting bone health and muscle maintenance for women over 60. Both turmeric and ginger are well-known for their anti-inflammatory effects, which can effectively alleviate joint discomfort and contribute to an overall improvement in health.

(Ready in: 30 minutes | Cook Duration: 20 minutes | Persons: 12 muffins)

Necessary Items:

- Almond flour: 2 cups
- Eggs: 3 large
- Coconut oil (melted): 1/4 cup
- Honey or maple syrup: 1/4 cup
- Ground turmeric: 1 tsp
- Ground ginger: 1 tsp
- Baking soda: 1/2 tsp
- Salt: 1/4 tsp
- Vanilla extract: 1 tsp

How to Prepare: Warm up the oven to 350 deg.F (175 deg.C), and line a muffin tray with paper liners. A big bowl should be used to combine the almond flour, ginger, turmeric, baking soda, and salt by whisking them together. Eggs, honey, melted coconut oil, and vanilla extract should be whisked together in a separate dish until they are completely smooth. To ensure that the wet and dry components are well blended, slowly incorporate the wet with the dry.

The batter should be poured into the muffin tin that has been prepared, with each cup being approximately three quarters full. In order to ensure that a toothpick placed into the middle of a muffin comes out clean, bake the muffins for 18 to 20 minutes. Wait 10 minutes prior to presenting the muffins so that they can cool down.

Nutritional Info: Calories: 150 kcal, Protein: 5g, Carbohydrates: 10g, Fat: 11g, Fiber: 2g, Sugars: 5g, Sodium: 90mg

20. Anti-Inflammatory Smoothie with Mango, Turmeric, and Spinach

This refreshing smoothie is loaded with anti-inflammatory ingredients like turmeric, spinach, and mango. Mango provides vitamin C for immune support, while turmeric and spinach help fight inflammation and promote healthy aging.

(Ready in: 5 minutes | Cook Duration: None | Persons: 2)

Ingredients:

- Fresh or frozen mango chunks: 1 cup
- Fresh spinach: 1 cup
- Coconut milk (unsweetened): 1 cup
- Ground turmeric: 1/2 tsp
- Fresh ginger (grated): 1/2 tsp
- Chia seeds: 1 tbsp
- Ice cubes (optional): 1/2 cup
- Honey or maple syrup (optional): 1 tbsp

Instructions: Add the mango, spinach, coconut milk, turmeric, ginger, chia seeds, and ice cubes (if using) to a mixer. Puree till it is silky smooth and creamy. If you want your smoothie to be sweeter, taste it and perhaps include some honey or maple syrup. Right away, present in glasses, and take pleasure in it.

Nutritional Info: Calories: 180 kcal, Protein: 3g, Carbohydrates: 29g, Fat: 8g, Fiber: 5g, Sugars: 17g, Sodium: 60mg

Chapter 7: Anti-Inflammatory Lunch Recipes

1.Quinoa Salad with Avocado, Kale, and Pomegranate

This vibrant quinoa salad is packed with nutrient-dense ingredients that support an anti-inflammatory diet. Quinoa provides complete protein, while avocado offers heart-healthy fats and kale delivers a wealth of vitamins. The addition of pomegranate seeds adds a refreshing burst of antioxidants, crucial for fighting inflammation. This recipe is ideal for women over 60, as it promotes heart health, supports bone strength, and aids digestion.

(Ready in: 15 mins | Cook Duration: 15 mins | Persons: 2)

Necessary Items:

- Quinoa: 1/2 cup (uncooked)
- Kale: 1 cup (severed)
- Avocado: 1 ripe, cubed
- Pomegranate seeds: 1/4 cup
- Olive oil: 2 tbsps
- Lemon juice: 1 tbsp
- Salt and pepper: as required
- Walnuts: 2 tbsps (optional, for crunch)

How to Prepare: In most cases, the quinoa should be cooked for around fifteen minutes, as specified on the package. Let it cool down. Combine the quinoa that has been cooked with the severed kale in a big bowl. The salad should be tossed to incorporate the lemon juice and olive oil that has been drizzled over it. In order to prevent the avocado from becoming mashed, include the chopped avocado and pomegranate seeds and mix them together carefully. Use salt and pepper as required, and flavor with salt, and sprinkle with walnuts if desired. Present instantly or chill in the fridge for a refreshing meal.

Nutritional Info: Calories: 320 kcal, Protein: 8g, Carbohydrates: 30g, Fat: 20g, Fiber: 8g, Vitamin C: 40% RDA, Iron: 10% RDA

2. Grilled Salmon with Turmeric-Spiced Lentils

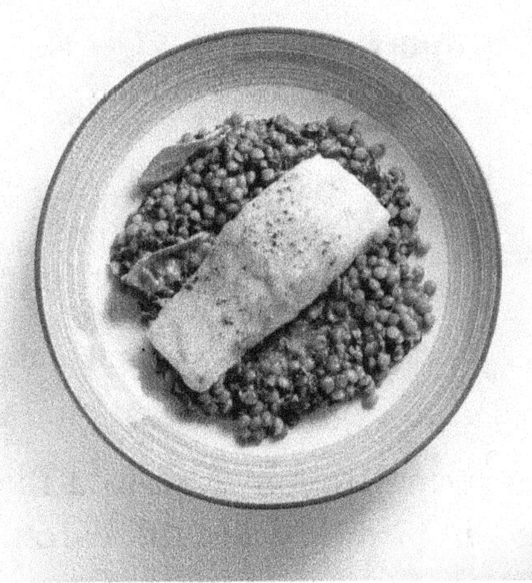

Salmon, rich in omega-3 fatty acids, is a powerful anti-inflammatory food that benefits cardiovascular health, making it ideal for women over 60. Paired with turmeric-spiced lentils, this meal offers a protein-rich, fiber-packed dish that promotes joint health and reduces inflammation.

(Prep Time: 10 mins | Cook time: 30min Persons: 2)

Necessary Items:

- Salmon fillets: 2 (about 4 oz each)
- Olive oil: 2 tbsps
- Lemon juice: 1 tbsp
- Lentils: 1 cup (uncooked)
- Turmeric powder: 1 tsp
- Garlic: 2 pieces (crushed)
- Onion: 1 small (severed)
- Spinach: 1 cup (fresh, severed)
- Salt and pepper: as required

How to Prepare: In most cases, the quinoa should be cooked for around 15 minutes, as specified on the package. Let it cool down. Combine the quinoa that has been cooked with the severed kale in a big bowl. The salad should be tossed to incorporate the lemon juice and olive oil that has been drizzled over it. In order to prevent the avocado from becoming mashed, include the chopped avocado and pomegranate seeds and mix them together carefully. Use pepper and salt as needed , and flavor with salt.

Nutritional Info: Calories: 460 kcal, Protein: 35g, Carbohydrates: 20g, Fat: 25g, Omega-3: 1,200mg, Fiber: 10g

3. Chickpea and Spinach Stew with Coconut Milk

This hearty stew combines the anti-inflammatory gains of chickpeas and spinach with the creamy texture of coconut milk. Chickpeas are an excellent source of fiber and plant-based protein, supporting gut health, while spinach provides essential vitamins and antioxidants. This comforting dish is perfect for women over 60, promoting digestive health and helping to manage blood sugar levels.

(Ready in: 10 minutes | Cook Duration: 25 minutes | Persons: 2)

Ingredients:

- Chickpeas: 1 can (15 oz), drained and rinsed
- Spinach: 2 cups (fresh, severed)
- Coconut milk: 1 cup (unsweetened)
- Olive oil: 1 tbsp
- Onion: 1 small (severed)
- Garlic: 2 pieces (crushed)
- Ginger: 1 tbsp (fresh, grated)
- Cumin powder: 1 tsp
- Turmeric powder: 1/2 tsp
- Salt and pepper: as required

Instructions: In a big saucepan, bring the olive oil to a middling temp. The severed onion, garlic, and ginger should be added and sautéed until the aroma is released. In order to release the flavors, stir in the cumin and turmeric and continue cooking for a minute. Gently whisk in the chickpeas and coconut milk until they are thoroughly combined. For around 10 minutes, allow the mixture to simmer in order to thicken. Proceed to cook the fresh spinach for an additional 3 to 4 minutes, until it has wilted. Add salt and pepper as required, and flavor with salt. Present the stew hot, optionally with brown rice or quinoa.

Nutritional Info: Calories: 320 kcal, Protein: 12g, Carbohydrates: 35g, Fat: 15g, Fiber: 10g, Vitamin A: 70% RDA, Iron: 25% RDA

4. Sweet Potato and Black Bean Tacos with Avocado Salsa

These sweet potato and black bean tacos are a delicious plant-based option packed with fiber and antioxidants. Sweet potatoes are rich in beta-carotene, which supports skin health and immunity, while black beans provide plant-based protein and help regulate blood sugar. The avocado salsa adds healthy fats, perfect for reducing inflammation and supporting heart health in women over 60.

(Ready in: 10 mins | Cook Duration: 25 mins | Persons: 2)

Necessary Items:

- Sweet potatoes: 1 large (skinned and cubed)
- Black beans: 1 can (15 oz), drained and rinsed
- Olive oil: 2 tbsps
- Cumin: 1 tsp
- Smoked paprika: 1 tsp
- Garlic powder: 1/2 tsp
- Corn tortillas: 4
- Avocado: 1 (cubed)
- Red onion: 1/4 (severed)
- Lime juice: 1 tbsp
- Fresh cilantro: 2 tbsps (severed)
- Salt and pepper: as required

How to Prepare: Warm up the oven to 400 deg.F (200 deg.C). A mixture of cumin, smoked paprika, garlic powder, salt, and pepper should be added to the sweet potatoes that have been cubed and then tossed. Put them on a baking sheet and roast them for 20 to 25 minutes, or until they are soft. During the time that the sweet potatoes are roasting, you may make the avocado salsa by putting in a small bowl cubed avocado, red onion, lime juice, fresh cilantro, and a little bit of salt. Black beans should be heated in a pot at middling temp. until they are completely warmed through. A dry skillet should be used to warm the corn tortillas for approximately thirty seconds on all sides. By layering the roasted sweet potatoes, black beans, and other ingredients, assemble the tacos, and avocado salsa on each tortilla. Present immediately, garnished with extra cilantro and lime wedges.

Nutritional Info: Calories: 380 kcal, Protein: 12g, Carbohydrates: 60g, Fat: 14g, Fiber: 15g, Vitamin A: 180% RDA, Iron: 20% RDA

5. Grilled Shrimp Salad with Arugula and Citrus Vinaigrette

This light and refreshing shrimp salad combines the lean protein of shrimp with the peppery bite of arugula and a tangy citrus vinaigrette. Shrimp is a great source of anti-inflammatory omega-3 fatty acids, while arugula is rich in vitamin K, supporting bone health. This salad is perfect for women over 60 looking for a low-calorie, nutrient-packed meal to support an anti-inflammatory diet.

(Prep Time: 10 minutes | Cook Time: 10 minutes | Servings: 2)

Ingredients:

- Shrimp: 12 medium (skinned and deveined)
- Arugula: 2 cups (fresh)
- Olive oil: 2 tbsps
- Orange juice: 2 tbsps (freshly squeezed)
- Lemon juice: 1 tbsp
- Dijon mustard: 1 tsp
- Garlic: 1 piece (crushed)
- Red onion: 1/4 (finely cut)
- Avocado: 1/2 (sliced)
- Salt and pepper: as required

Instructions: A grill pan should be heated at a middling temp. When the shrimp are ready, flavor them with salt and pepper and drizzle them with olive oil. The shrimp should be grilled for 2 to 3 minutes on all sides, or until they are pink and opaque. When you want to make citrus vinaigrette, put the olive oil, orange juice, lemon juice, Dijon mustard, smashed garlic, salt, and pepper into a small bowl and whisk all of the ingredients together. The citrus vinaigrette should be mixed with the fresh arugula and the chunks of red onion that are placed in a big bowl. Top the salad with grilled shrimp and avocado pieces. Present immediately, garnished with additional citrus pieces if desired.

Nutritional Info: Calories: 280 kcal, Protein: 20g, Carbohydrates: 12g, Fat: 18g, Omega-3: 500mg, Fiber: 4g, Vitamin C: 60% RDA

6. Cauliflower Rice Bowl with Tofu and Ginger-Sesame Dressing

This cauliflower rice bowl with tofu and ginger-sesame dressing is a low-carb, anti-inflammatory meal that's rich in plant-based protein and healthy fats. Cauliflower is packed with fiber and antioxidants, while tofu provides a great source of protein, especially for women over 60 who are looking to reduce inflammation and support muscle mass.

(Ready in: 10 mins | Cook Duration: 20 mins | Persons: 2)

Necessary Items:

- Cauliflower: 1 small head (grated into rice-like pieces)
- Firm tofu: 1 block (cubed)
- Olive oil: 2 tbsps
- Soy sauce: 2 tbsps
- Sesame oil: 1 tbsp
- Fresh ginger: 1 tbsp (grated)
- Garlic: 1 piece (crushed)

- Rice vinegar: 1 tbsp
- Sesame seeds: 1 tbsp
- Green onions: 2 (severed)
- Carrots: 1 (shredded)
- Cucumber: 1 (sliced)
- Salt and pepper: as required

How to Prepare: A grill pan should be heated at middling temp. When the shrimp are ready, flavor them with salt and pepper and drizzle them with olive oil. The shrimp should be grilled for 2 to 3 minutes on all sides, or until they are pink and opaque. When you want to form the citrus vinaigrette, put the olive oil, orange juice, lemon juice, Dijon mustard, smashed garlic, salt, and pepper into a small bowl and whisk all of the ingredients together. The citrus vinaigrette should be mixed with the fresh arugula and the chunks of red onion that are placed in a big bowl. Assemble the bowls by layering the cauliflower rice, cooked tofu, shredded carrots, and sliced cucumber. The ginger-sesame sauce should be drizzled over the top, and green onions and crushed sesame seeds should be used as garnishes.

Nutritional Info: Calories: 290 kcal, Protein: 16g, Carbohydrates: 18g, Fat: 18g, Fiber: 7g, Vitamin C: 60% RDA, Calcium: 15% RDA

7. Turmeric-Spiced Chicken Wrap with Cucumber and Hummus

This turmeric-spiced chicken wrap is a flavorful, anti-inflammatory lunch option that's rich in lean protein and healthy fats. Turmeric helps to reduce inflammation, while the hummus and cucumber add a refreshing crunch.

(Ready in: 10 minutes | Cook Duration: 15 minutes | Persons: 2)

Necessary Items:

- Chicken breast: 1 big (cut into strips)
- Turmeric: 1 tsp
- Paprika: 1/2 tsp
- Olive oil: 1 tbsp
- Whole wheat wraps: 2
- Hummus: 1/4 cup
- Cucumber: 1 (finely cut)
- Baby spinach: 1 cup
- Lemon juice: 1 tbsp
- Salt and pepper: as required

How to Prepare: Put the olive oil, turmeric, paprika, salt, and pepper into a bowl and stir them together. The chicken strips should be coated by tossing them in the mixture. To ensure that the chicken strips are cooked through, warm a skillet at middling temp. and cook them for approximately 5 to 7 minutes on all sides. A dry skillet should be used to warm the wraps made from whole wheat for around 30 seconds. First, spread hummus on each wrap in a uniform layer, and then pile on spinach, cucumber slices, and chicken that has been seasoned with turmeric. Drizzle with lemon juice, fold the wraps, and serve immediately.

Nutritional Info: Calories: 340 kcal, Protein: 28g, Carbohydrates: 30g, Fat: 13g, Fiber: 7g, Vitamin A: 35% RDA, Iron: 10% RDA

8. Roasted Beet and Goat Cheese Salad with Walnuts

This roasted beet and goat cheese salad is a nutrient-dense, anti-inflammatory meal loaded with antioxidants. Beets are high in nitrates, supporting heart health, while goat cheese provides healthy fats and a creamy texture. Walnuts add a boost of omega-3s, making this a perfect lunch for women over 60 to support brain health and reduce inflammation.

(Prep Time: 10 minutes | Cook Time: 45 minutes | Servings: 2)

Ingredients:

- Beets: 2 medium (trimmed and scrubbed)
- Olive oil: 2 tbsps
- Goat cheese: 2 oz. (crumbled)
- Walnuts: 1/4 cup (toasted)
- Mixed greens: 2 cups
- Balsamic vinegar: 1 tbsp
- Honey: 1 tsp
- Salt and pepper: as required

Instructions: Warm up oven to 400 deg.F (200 deg.C). Wrap the beets in aluminum foil and roast for 40-45 minutes until tender. After allowing them to cool, peel and slice them. To make the dressing, blend the honey, balsamic vinegar, olive oil, and salt & pepper in a small bowl and mix all of the components together. The mixed greens should be arranged on a platter, and then roasted beet slices, crumbled goat cheese, and toasted walnuts should be placed on top of the greens. After the balsamic dressing has been drizzled over the salad, it should be served right away.

Nutritional Info: Calories: 320 kcal, Protein: 8g, Carbohydrates: 22g, Fat: 24g, Fiber: 6g, Omega-3: 500mg, Vitamin C: 25% RDA

9. Quinoa and Grilled Vegetable Buddha Bowl with Tahini Dressing

This quinoa and grilled vegetable Buddha bowl is packed with plant-based protein, fiber, and healthy fats. Quinoa is a complete protein that supports muscle maintenance, while grilled vegetables and tahini dressing add essential nutrients and antioxidants, making this dish ideal for women over 60 looking to reduce inflammation.

(Ready in: 15 min | Cook Duration: 25 min | Persons: 2)

Necessary Items:

- Quinoa: 1 cup (cooked)
- Zucchini: 1 (sliced)
- Red bell pepper: 1 (sliced)
- Eggplant: 1/2 (sliced)
- Olive oil: 2 tbsps
- Tahini: 2 tbsps
- Lemon juice: 1 tbsp
- Garlic: 1 piece (crushed)
- Water: 2 tbsps
- Salt and pepper: as required

How to Prepare: A grill pan should be heated at a middling temp. Olive oil, salt, and pepper should be mixed with pieces of zucchini, red bell pepper, and eggplant before being assembled. The vegetables should be grilled for 3 to 4 minutes on all sides until they are browned and soft. In order to make the tahini dressing, combine the tahini, lemon juice, minced garlic, water, salt, and pepper in a small bowl and whisk every one of the components together. Assemble the Buddha bowls by layering cooked quinoa and grilled vegetables. Drizzle with tahini dressing and serve immediately.

Nutritional Info: Calories: 400 kcal, Protein: 12g, Carbohydrates: 50g, Fat: 20g, Fiber: 10g, Magnesium: 30% RDA, Iron: 15% RDA

10. Grilled Turkey Burgers with Avocado and Spinach

These grilled turkey burgers are a lean source of protein, combined with heart-healthy avocado and nutrient-rich spinach. Perfect for women over 60, this meal supports muscle health and offers anti-inflammatory benefits thanks to the combination of ingredients like avocado and olive oil.

(Prep Time: 10 minutes | Cook Time: 15 minutes | Servings: 2)

Ingredients:

- Ground turkey: 1/2 pound
- Olive oil: 1 tbsp
- Garlic powder: 1/2 tsp
- Onion powder: 1/2 tsp
- Whole wheat buns: 2
- Avocado: 1 (sliced)
- Fresh spinach: 1 cup
- Salt and pepper: as required

Instructions: The ground turkey, garlic powder, onion powder, salt, and pepper should be mixed together in a basin or bowl. The components should be formed into two patties. Olive oil should be brushed onto a grill or grill pan before it is heated at a middling temp. To ensure that the turkey burgers are completely cooked, grill them for five to six minutes on all sides. Toast the whole wheat buns on the grill for about 1 minute. Assemble the burgers by layering spinach, grilled turkey patties, and avocado pieces on each bun.

Nutritional Info: Calories: 370 kcal, Protein: 32g, Carbohydrates: 25g, Fat: 18g, Fiber: 6g, Vitamin A: 20% RDA, Potassium: 500mg

11. Tuna Salad with Avocado and Cucumber on Mixed Greens

This tuna salad combines the healthy fats from avocado with protein-rich tuna, making it a nutrient-dense meal for women over 60. The avocado supports heart health, while tuna provides lean protein and omega-3 fatty acids, perfect for reducing inflammation and supporting joint and cognitive health.

(Prep Time: 10 minutes | Cook Time: None | Servings: 2)

Ingredients:

- Canned tuna (in water, drained): 1 can   (about 5 oz.)

- Avocado: 1 (cubed)
- Cucumber: 1 (sliced)
- Mixed greens: 2 cups
- Olive oil: 1 tbsp
- Lemon juice: 1 tbsp
- Salt and pepper: as required
- Cherry tomatoes (optional): 1/2 cup (halved)

Instructions: To make the tuna salad, combine the tuna that has been drained, severed avocado, and sliced cucumber in a bowl. To prepare a dressing, take a distinct, smaller bowl and blend the olive oil, lemon juice, salt, and pepper by whisking them together. Put mixed greens on two plates and top with the tuna, avocado, and cucumber mixture. Drizzle with the lemon dressing, and add cherry tomatoes if desired.

Nutritional Info: Calories: 320 kcal, Protein: 28g, Carbohydrates: 12g, Fat: 20g, Fiber: 7g, Omega-3: 900mg, Vitamin C: 35% RDA

12. Chickpea and Cucumber Salad with Lemon-Tahini Dressing

This chickpea and cucumber salad is a refreshing, plant-based option that provides fiber, protein, and healthy fats. Chickpeas are an excellent source of plant-based protein and fiber, which helps maintain healthy digestion. The tahini dressing adds a rich, nutty flavor with anti-inflammatory benefits, making it ideal for women over 60.

(Ready in: 10 minutes | Cook Duration: None | Persons: 2)

Necessary Items:

- Canned chickpeas (drained and washed): 1 cup
- Cucumber: 1 (sliced)
- Red onion: 1/4 (finely cut)
- Fresh parsley: 1/4 cup (severed)
- Lemon juice: 2 tbsps
- Tahini: 1 tbsp
- Olive oil: 1 tbsp
- Garlic: 1 piece (crushed)
- Salt and pepper: as required

How to Prepare: The chickpeas, sliced cucumber, red onion, and severed parsley should be mixed together in a separate big basin. The dressing is made by combining lemon juice, tahini, olive oil, chopped garlic, salt, and pepper in a small bowl and whisking all of the components together. To ensure that the chickpea mixture is uniformly coated, pour the dressing over it and toss it. Can be served either chilled or at room temp.

Nutritional Info: Calories: 290 kcal, Protein: 10g, Carbohydrates: 28g, Fat: 14g, Fiber: 8g, Vitamin A: 15% RDA, Iron: 20% RDA

13. Baked Cod with Herb-Infused Quinoa and Asparagus

Baked cod is a lean, protein-rich fish that pairs beautifully with herb-infused quinoa and asparagus. This dish is packed with omega-3 fatty acids, lean protein, and anti-inflammatory ingredients, making it perfect for women over 60 who want to support cardiovascular health and maintain lean muscle mass.

(Ready in: 10 minutes | Cook Duration: 20 minutes| Persons: 2)

Necessary Items:

- Cod fillets: 2 (about 4 oz. each)
- Olive oil: 2 tbsps
- Fresh herbs (parsley, thyme): 2 tbsps (severed)
- Quinoa: 1 cup (cooked)
- Asparagus: 8 spears (trimmed)
- Lemon: 1 (sliced)
- Garlic: 1 piece (crushed)
- Salt and pepper: as required

How to Prepare: Warm up the oven to 375 deg.F (190 deg.C). The cod fillets should be placed on a baking pan that has been lined with parchment paper. To finish, drizzle with olive oil, sprinkle with severed herbs, garlic, salt, and pepper, then finish with slices of lemon. Fish should be baked for 15 to 20 minutes, or until it can be readily flaked with a fork. In the meantime, prepare the quinoa in accordance with the instructions on the package, and steam the asparagus for 5 to 7 minutes, until it is soft. Present the baked cod on top of quinoa that has been flavored with herbs, and serve steamed asparagus on the side.

Nutritional Info: Calories: 350 kcal, Protein: 32g, Carbohydrates: 30g, Fat: 10g, Fiber: 5g, Omega-3: 500mg, Vitamin C: 40% RDA

14. Red Lentil and Sweet Potato Curry with Spinach

This red lentil and sweet potato curry is a warm, hearty dish packed with plant-based protein and fiber. The sweet potatoes and spinach add essential vitamins and minerals, while the spices help reduce inflammation. This meal is ideal for women over 60 who want to support heart health and improve digestion.

(Ready in: 10 minutes | Cook Duration: 25 minutes | Persons: 2)

Necessary Items:

- Red lentils: 1 cup (rinsed)
- Sweet potato: 1 large (skinned and cubed)
- Coconut milk: 1 cup
- Fresh spinach: 2 cups
- Onion: 1 small (cubed)
- Garlic: 2 pieces (crushed)
- Curry powder: 1 tbsp
- Turmeric: 1 tsp
- Olive oil: 1 tbsp
- Salt and pepper: as required

How to Prepare: In a big saucepan, bring the olive oil to a middling temp. For 3 to 4 minutes, make sure the crushed garlic and cubed onion are softened by sautéing them. Cook for a further 2 to 3 minutes after adding the cubed sweet potato, curry powder, turmeric, salt, and pepper from the seasonings. Add the red lentils and coconut milk and stir to blend. To ensure that the lentils and sweet potato are cooked through, bring the mixture to a simmer and continue cooking for 20 to 25 minutes. For around 2 minutes, stir in the fresh spinach until it has wilted. Present the curry hot.

Nutritional Info: Calories: 420 kcal, Protein: 18g, Carbohydrates: 58g, Fat: 14g, Fiber: 16g, Vitamin A: 150% RDA, Iron: 25% RDA

15. Grilled Chicken Salad with Mixed Berries and Walnuts

This grilled chicken salad combines lean protein with antioxidant-rich berries and heart-healthy walnuts. Berries are known for their anti-inflammatory properties, while walnuts provide omega-3 fatty acids. This balanced meal is perfect for women over 60 looking to maintain a healthy weight and support cognitive function.

(Ready in: 10 minutes | Cook Duration: 15 minutes | Persons: 2)

Necessary Items:

- Chicken breast: 1 large (grilled and sliced)
- Mixed greens: 2 cups
- Mixed berries (blueberries, strawberries, raspberries): 1 cup
- Walnuts: 1/4 cup (toasted)
- Olive oil: 2 tbsps
- Balsamic vinegar: 1 tbsp
- Dijon mustard: 1 tsp
- Salt and pepper: as required

How to Prepare: To ensure that the chicken breast is completely done, grill it for 6 to 8 minutes on all sides, and then slice it very finely. To prepare the dressing, blend the olive oil, balsamic vinegar, Dijon mustard, salt, and pepper in a small bowl and whisk all of the components together. Arrange mixed greens on two plates and top with grilled chicken pieces, mixed berries, and toasted walnuts. Drizzle with the balsamic dressing and serve immediately.

Nutritional Info: Calories: 400 kcal, Protein: 30g, Carbohydrates: 18g, Fat: 25g, Fiber: 6g, Vitamin C: 50% RDA, Omega-3: 600mg

16. Roasted Carrot and Parsnip Soup with Ginger

This roasted carrot and parsnip soup is a comforting and nutrient-packed dish. Carrots and parsnips are rich in antioxidants and fiber, while ginger adds anti-inflammatory benefits. This soup is perfect for women over 60, promoting digestion and supporting overall immune health.

(Ready in: 10 minutes | Cook Duration: 35 minutes | Persons: 2)

Necessary Items:

- Carrots: 4 (skinned and severed)
- Parsnips: 2 (skinned and severed)
- Fresh ginger: 1 tbsp (grated)
- Olive oil: 2 tbsps
- Onion: 1 small (cubed)
- Garlic: 2 pieces (crushed)
- Vegetable broth: 4 cups
- Salt and pepper: as required
- Fresh parsley (optional): for garnish

How to Prepare: Warm up the oven to 400 deg.F (200 deg.C). Arrange the carrots and parsnips that have been severed on a baking sheet, drizzle them with 1 tbsp of olive oil, and roast them for 25 to 30 minutes, or until they are soft. The rest of the olive oil should be heated in a big saucepan, and then the chopped onion and crushed garlic should be sautéed for 3 to 4 minutes, until they become tender. Add the roasted carrots, parsnips, grated ginger, and vegetable broth to the pot. Simmer for 10 minutes. Use an immersion blender to blend the soup until smooth. Season with salt and pepper as required. Present hot, garnished with fresh parsley if desired.

Nutritional Info: Calories: 220 kcal, Protein: 4g, Carbohydrates: 40g, Fat: 8g, Fiber: 8g, Vitamin A: 300% RDA, Vitamin C: 35% RDA

17. Spinach and Mushroom Frittata with Sweet Potatoes

This spinach and mushroom frittata offers a combination of lean protein and fiber with nutrient-dense vegetables. The addition of sweet potatoes provides complex carbohydrates, making it a satisfying meal for women over 60 who need to maintain steady energy levels and reduce inflammation.

(Ready in: 10 minutes | Cook Duration: 25 minutes | Persons: 2)

Necessary Items:

- Eggs: 4
- Spinach: 2 cups (fresh)
- Mushrooms: 1 cup (sliced)
- Sweet potato: 1 small (skinned and cubed)
- Olive oil: 1 tbsp
- Onion: 1/2 (cubed)
- Garlic: 1 piece (crushed)
- Salt and pepper: as required
- Fresh herbs (optional): for garnish

How to Prepare: Warm up the oven to 375 deg.F (190 deg.C). In a skillet that can go in the oven, warm the olive oil at middling temp. Then, sauté the sweet potato dice for 5 to 7 minutes, or until it is just little soft. Cook for an additional 4 to 5 minutes after adding the severed onion, garlic, and sliced mushrooms. This will allow the vegetables to become more tender. Fresh spinach should be stirred in and cooked until it has wilted. Place the eggs in a distinct bowl and mix them with the salt and pepper. Over the vegetables that are already in the skillet, pour the eggs. After placing the skillet in the oven, bake the frittata for 12 to 15 minutes, or until it has reached the desired consistency. Present warm, garnished with fresh herbs if desired.

Nutritional Info: Calories: 280 kcal, Protein: 15g, Carbohydrates: 22g, Fat: 15g, Fiber: 6g, Vitamin A: 120% RDA, Iron: 15% RDA

18. Black Bean and Quinoa Stuffed Zucchini Boats

These black bean and quinoa stuffed zucchini boats are a flavorful, plant-based dish rich in protein and fiber. Black beans and quinoa make this meal ideal for supporting muscle mass and reducing inflammation in women over 60, while zucchini provides essential vitamins and minerals.

(Ready in: 10 minutes | Cook Duration: 25 minutes | Persons: 2)

Necessary Items:

- Zucchini: 2 large (halved and scooped out)
- Black beans: 1/2 cup (cooked)
- Quinoa: 1/2 cup (cooked)
- Tomato: 1 small (cubed)
- Red bell pepper: 1/2 (cubed)
- Olive oil: 1 tbsp
- Garlic: 1 piece (crushed)
- Cumin: 1 tsp
- Salt and pepper: as required
- Fresh cilantro (optional): for garnish

How to Prepare: Warm up the oven to 375 deg.F (190 deg.C). After halving the zucchinis, drizzle them with olive oil and bake them in the oven for 10 to 15 minutes, or until they are soft. To sauté the garlic, cubed tomato, and bell pepper for 3 to 4 minutes, warm the rest of the olive oil in a skillet at middling temp. Stir the mixture occasionally. The cooked black beans, quinoa, cumin, salt, and pepper should be stirred in at this point. Cook for 2 to 3 minutes, until everything is thoroughly blended. Bake the zucchini halves for a further 10 minutes after spooning the mixture into the halves that have been roasted. Fresh cilantro should be used as a garnish prior to presenting.

Nutritional Info: Calories: 320 kcal, Protein: 14g, Carbohydrates: 40g, Fat: 12g, Fiber: 10g, Vitamin C: 80% RDA, Iron: 20% RDA

19. Salmon Salad with Mixed Greens and Lemon-Tahini Dressing

This salmon salad combines omega-3-rich salmon with mixed greens and a creamy lemon-tahini dressing. Salmon supports heart and brain health, making this dish perfect for women over 60. The dressing adds a rich source of healthy fats, essential for reducing inflammation.

(Ready in: 10 minutes | Cook Duration: 15 minutes | Persons: 2)

Necessary Items:

- Salmon fillet: 1 large (grilled or baked)
- Mixed greens: 2 cups
- Cherry tomatoes: 1/2 cup (halved)
- Cucumber: 1/2 (sliced)
- Avocado: 1/2 (sliced)
- Lemon juice: 2 tbsps
- Tahini: 1 tbsp
- Olive oil: 1 tbsp
- Salt and pepper: as required

How to Prepare: Grill or bake the salmon fillet for 12-15 minutes until fully cooked. Let cool slightly, then flake the salmon into pieces. To prepare the dressing, combine the lemon juice, tahini, olive oil, salt, and pepper in a small bowl and whisk every one of the components together. Organize mixed greens on two plates and top with cherry tomatoes, cucumber pieces, avocado, and flaked salmon. The salad should be served instantly after the lemon-tahini dressing has been drizzled over it.

Nutritional Info: Calories: 400 kcal, Protein: 30g, Carbohydrates: 12g, Fat: 28g, Omega-3: 1100mg, Vitamin A: 50% RDA, Iron: 15% RDA

20. Roasted Chickpea and Avocado Wrap with Turmeric Hummus

This roasted chickpea and avocado wrap is a satisfying, plant-based meal full of fiber, healthy fats, and anti-inflammatory properties. The turmeric hummus adds extra benefits, making it ideal for women over 60 who are looking to reduce joint pain and inflammation.

(Ready in: 10 minutes | Cook Duration: 20 minutes | Persons: 2)

Necessary Items:

For the Main Dish:

- Chickpeas: 1 cup (cooked and drained)
- Avocado: 1 (sliced)
- Whole-grain wraps: 2
- Turmeric hummus: 1/4 cup
- Olive oil: 1 tbsp
- Salt and pepper: as required
- Lemon juice: 1 tbsp
- Mixed greens: 1 cup
- Garlic powder: 1/2 tsp
- Paprika: 1/2 tsp

How to Prepare: Warm up the oven to 400 deg.F (200 deg.C). Using olive oil, garlic powder, paprika, salt, and pepper, toss the chickpeas that have been cooked. Then, roast them on a baking sheet for 15 to 20 minutes, or until they become crispy. Spread turmeric hummus over the whole-grain wraps and top with roasted chickpeas, avocado pieces, mixed greens, and a squeeze of lemon juice. Roll the wraps tightly and slice in half before serving.

Nutritional Info: Calories: 360 kcal, Protein: 12g, Carbohydrates: 40g, Fat: 18g, Fiber: 10g, Vitamin C: 30% RDA, Iron: 15% RDA

Chapter 8: Anti-Inflammatory Dinner Recipes

1. Baked Salmon with Garlic and Rosemary Sweet Potatoes

This dish is packed with omega-3 fatty acids from salmon, which are known for their anti-inflammatory properties, making it perfect for women over 60 aiming to reduce inflammation. Combined with nutrient-dense sweet potatoes rich in fiber and antioxidants, this meal supports heart health, boosts immunity, and helps maintain healthy skin and joints.

(Prep Time: 40mins | Cook Time: 30mins | Serves: 2)

Ingredients:

- Salmon fillets: 2 (about 6 oz each)
- Sweet potatoes: 2 medium, cut into wedges
- Fresh rosemary: 1 tbsp, finely severed
- Garlic: 3 pieces, crushed
- Olive oil: 2 tbsps
- Lemon: 1, sliced
- Sea salt: 1/2 tsp
- Black pepper: 1/2 tsp

Instructions: Warm up your oven to 400 deg.F (200 deg.C). Put the sweet potato wedges in a big bowl and include 1 tbsp of olive oil, garlic, rosemary, salt, and pepper. Toss the mixture until the sweet potato wedges are uniformly covered. A single layer of sweet potatoes should be spread out on a baking sheet, and then they should be baked for 15 minutes. During the time that the sweet potatoes are in the oven, brush the salmon fillets with the rest of the olive oil and season them with salt and pepper. Lemon slices should be placed on top of each fillet before serving. Once the sweet potatoes have been in the oven for 15 minutes, take them out from the oven and distribute them on one side of the baking sheet. Position the salmon fillets on the opposite side of the pan. Put the baking sheet back into the oven and continue baking for an extra 15 minutes, or until the salmon is fully cooked and the sweet potatoes have reached a golden brown color and are soft. Present the baked salmon with the roasted sweet potatoes and enjoy.

Nutritional Info: Calories: 450 kcal, Protein: 30g, Carbohydrates: 28g, Fat: 24g, Saturated Fat: 4g, Cholesterol: 70mg, Sodium: 320mg, Potassium: 950mg, Sugars: 8g

2. Lentil and Vegetable Shepherd's Pie

This plant-based version of a classic shepherd's pie is loaded with lentils and vegetables, making it a high-fiber, nutrient-rich meal that supports gut health and reduces inflammation. Perfect for women over 60, lentils are a great source of plant protein, while the mix of vegetables provides essential vitamins and minerals.

(Ready in: 1 hour | Cook Duration: 45 minutes | Persons: 4)

Necessary Items:

- Green or brown lentils: 1 cup, dried
- Vegetable broth: 2 cups
- Carrots: 2, cubed
- Onion: 1, severed

- Celery stalks: 2, cubed
- Garlic: 2 pieces, crushed
- Tomato paste: 2 tbsps
- Thyme: 1 tsp, dried
- Olive oil: 2 tbsps

- Mashed potatoes: 4 cups (prepared from boiled potatoes, mashed with olive oil or plant-based milk)
- Peas: 1/2 cup, frozen
- Salt: 1/2 tsp
- Black pepper: 1/2 tsp

How to Prepare: Warm up the oven to 375 deg.F (190 deg.F). In a medium pot, cook the lentils in vegetable broth according to package instructions (about 20 minutes). Once cooked, drain and set aside. Prepare the olive oil by heating it in a big skillet at middling temp. Garlic, onions, carrots, and celery should be sautéed for around 5 minutes, or until they become more tender. A mixture of tomato paste, thyme, salt, and pepper should be stirred in. Mix the lentils and peas that have been cooked until they are completely incorporated. Maintain a low simmer for 10 minutes with the mixture. Put the lentil-vegetable mixture into a casserole dish and smooth it out so that it is uniformly distributed. Put mashed potatoes on top, spreading them out to form a layer that is smooth. Bake the mashed potatoes for 25 to 30 minutes, or until they are golden brown and somewhat crispy. Prior to presenting, let the dish to cool for a couple of minutes.

Nutrition: Calories: 320 kcal, Protein: 12g, Carbohydrates: 48g, Fat: 9g, Saturated Fat: 1.5g, Cholesterol: 0mg, Sodium: 410mg, Potassium: 800mg, Sugars: 6g

3. Turmeric and Ginger Chicken Stir-Fry with Broccoli

This vibrant chicken stir-fry combines anti-inflammatory powerhouses like turmeric and ginger with broccoli, a cruciferous vegetable known for its cancer-fighting properties. It's a quick and flavorful dish that supports joint health and reduces inflammation, ideal for women over 60 looking to maintain vitality and energy.

(Ready in: 25 minutes | Cook Duration: 15mins | Serving 2)

Necessary Items:

- Boneless, skinless chicken breasts: 2, sliced into strips
- Broccoli florets: 2 cups
- Fresh ginger: 1 tbsp, grated
- Turmeric powder: 1 tsp
- Garlic: 2 pieces, crushed
- Soy sauce (or tamari for gluten-free): 2 tbsps

- Olive oil: 2 tbsps
- Lemon juice: 1 tbsp
- Sesame seeds: 1 tsp (optional, for garnish)
- Salt: 1/4 tsp
- Black pepper: 1/4 tsp

How to Prepare: Take a big skillet or wok and warm it at med-high temp. Include 1 tbsp of olive oil in the pan. Cook the chicken strips for approximately 5 to 7 minutes, or until they have a golden-brown color and are fully cooked. Take the food out of the skillet and put it away. After adding the rest of the olive oil to the same skillet, sauté the garlic, ginger, and turmeric for a minute, or until the aroma is released out of them. Stir-frying the broccoli florets for around 5 minutes, until they are bright green and slightly soft, is the recommended method of cooking.

Put the chicken that has been cooked back into the skillet, along with the lemon juice, soy sauce, salt, and pepper. Cook for another three minutes while stirring everything together until it is completely incorporated. The dish should be removed from the heat and topped with sesame seeds before being served.

Nutritional Info: Calories: 350 kcal, Protein: 35g, Carbohydrates: 10g, Fat: 18g, Saturated Fat: 3g, Cholesterol: 90mg, Sodium: 600mg, Potassium: 900mg, Sugars: 2g

4. Grilled Tofu with Sesame Spinach and Brown Rice

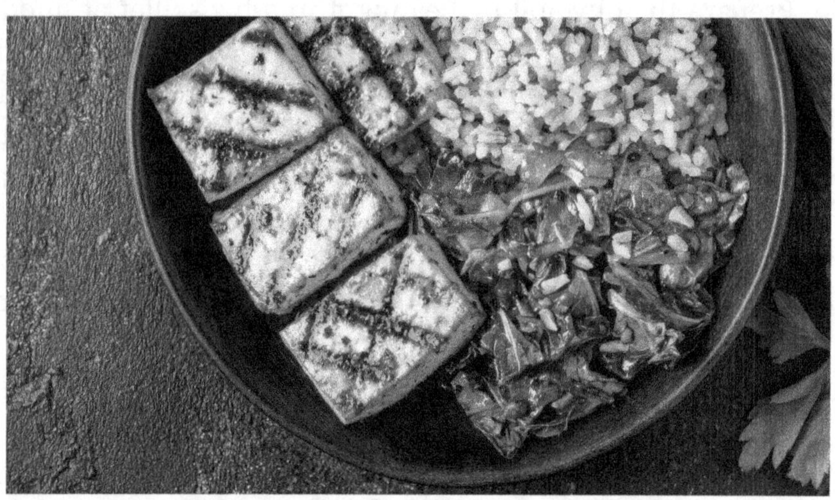

This plant-based dish is a nutritious, anti-inflammatory option for women over 60. Tofu provides a high-quality source of protein, while sesame seeds and spinach are packed with antioxidants, vitamins, and minerals that help support bone health, fight inflammation, and promote heart health. The fiber-rich brown rice rounds out the meal for sustained energy.

(Ready in: 30 mins | Cook Duration: 20 mins | Persons: 2)

Necessary Items:

- Firm tofu: 1 block (about 14 oz), drained and sliced into cubes
- Brown rice: 1 cup, uncooked
- Spinach: 4 cups, fresh
- Sesame seeds: 2 tbsps, toasted
- Soy sauce (or tamari for gluten-free): 2 tbsps
- Sesame oil: 1 tbsp
- Olive oil: 1 tbsp
- Garlic: 2 pieces, crushed
- Lemon juice: 1 tbsp
- Salt: 1/2 tsp
- Black pepper: 1/4 tsp

How to Prepare: To prepare the brown rice, cook it for approximately 20 minutes, as directed on the package. During the time that the rice is cooking, set a grill pan at med-high temp. and warm the olive oil. When the tofu cubes are brown and crispy, add them on the grill and cook them for 4 to 5 minutes on all sides. Take the food out of the pan and put it away. The garlic should be sautéed in the same pan for a minute until it becomes aromatic. The sesame oil should be heated. After adding the spinach, continue to boil it for another 2 to 3 minutes until it has wilted. Incorporate the lemon juice, sesame seeds, and soy sauce into the mixture.

Use pepper and salt to season the food. Present the grilled tofu over a bed of brown rice, topped with the sesame spinach. Garnish with additional sesame seeds if desired.

Nutritional Info: Calories: 410 kcal, Protein: 19g, Carbohydrates: 40g, Fat: 18g, Saturated Fat: 2.5g, Cholesterol: 0mg, Sodium: 620mg, Potassium: 800mg, Sugars: 1g

5. Wild-Caught Cod with Sautéed Spinach and Cherry Tomatoes

Cod is a lean source of protein that's also rich in omega-3 fatty acids, making it an excellent anti-inflammatory food for women over 60. Paired with nutrient-dense spinach and antioxidant-packed cherry tomatoes, this dish supports heart health, brain function, and overall well-being.

(Ready in: 25 minutes | Cook Duration: 15 minutes | Persons: 2)

Ingredients:

- Wild-caught cod fillets: 2 (about 6 oz each)
- Spinach: 4 cups, fresh
- Cherry tomatoes: 1 cup, halved
- Olive oil: 2 tbsps
- Garlic: 2 pieces, crushed
- Lemon: 1, cut into wedges
- Sea salt: 1/2 tsp
- Black pepper: 1/4 tsp
- Fresh parsley: 1 tbsp, severed (optional, for garnish)

Instructions: To prepare the brown rice, cook it for approximately 20 minutes, as directed on the package. During the time that the rice is cooking, set a grill pan at med-high temp. and warm the olive oil. When the tofu cubes are brown and crispy, add them on the grill and cook them for 4 to 5 minutes on all sides. Take the food out of the pan and put it away. The garlic should be sautéed in the same pan for a minute until it becomes aromatic. The sesame oil should be heated. After adding the spinach, continue to boil it for another 2 to 3 minutes until it has wilted. Incorporate the lemon juice, sesame seeds, and soy sauce into the mixture. Use pepper and salt to season the food.

Nutritional Info: Calories: 320 kcal, Protein: 32g, Carbohydrates: 8g, Fat: 16g, Saturated Fat: 2.5g, Cholesterol: 70mg, Sodium: 300mg, Potassium: 850mg, Sugars: 4g

6. Balsamic-Glazed Portobello Mushrooms with Zucchini Noodles

This satisfying vegetarian dish features balsamic-glazed portobello mushrooms, which are rich in antioxidants and anti-inflammatory compounds. Paired with zucchini noodles, it's a light, low-carb option that supports healthy digestion and provides essential nutrients, perfect for women over 60 following an anti-inflammatory diet.

(Ready in: 25mins | Cook Duration: 15mins | Persons: 2)

Necessary Items:

- Large portobello mushrooms: 2
- Zucchini: 2, spiralized into noodles
- Balsamic vinegar: 2 tbsps
- Olive oil: 2 tbsps

- Garlic: 2 pieces, crushed
- Fresh basil: 2 tbsps, severed
- Sea salt: 1/2 tsp
- Black pepper: 1/4 tsp
- Parmesan (optional): 1 tbsp, grated for garnish

How to Prepare: To prepare the brown rice, cook it for approximately 20 minutes, as directed on the package. During the time that the rice is cooking, set a grill pan at med-high temp. and warm the olive oil. When the tofu cubes are brown and crispy, add them on the grill and cook them for 4 to 5 minutes on all sides. Take the food out of the pan and put it away. The garlic should be sautéed in the same pan for a minute until it becomes aromatic. The sesame oil should be heated. After adding the spinach, continue to boil it for another 2 to 3 minutes until it has wilted. Incorporate the lemon juice, sesame seeds, and soy sauce into the mixture. Use pepper and salt to season the food. Present the roasted mushrooms over the zucchini noodles, garnished with fresh basil and optional grated Parmesan.

Nutritional Info: Calories: 190 kcal, Protein: 4g, Carbohydrates: 15g, Fat: 12g, Saturated Fat: 2g, Cholesterol: 0mg, Sodium: 290mg, Potassium: 700mg, Sugars: 9g

7. Coconut-Curry Shrimp with Cauliflower Rice

This flavorful dish combines anti-inflammatory coconut milk and curry spices with protein-packed shrimp, making it an ideal dinner for women over 60. The addition of cauliflower rice keeps it low in carbs, supporting weight management and digestive health.

(Ready in: 30 minutes | Cook Duration: 20 minutes | Persons: 2)

Necessary Items:

- Shrimp (skinned and deveined): 12 large
- Cauliflower: 1 small head, grated into rice
- Coconut milk (light): 1 cup
- Curry powder: 1 tbsp
- Coconut oil: 1 tbsp
- Garlic: 2 pieces, crushed
- Fresh ginger: 1 tbsp, grated
- Lime: 1, juiced
- Fresh cilantro: 2 tbsps, severed
- Sea salt: 1/2 tsp
- Black pepper: 1/4 tsp

How to Prepare: At middling temp., bring the coconut oil to a temperature in a big skillet. Garlic and ginger should be added and sautéed for a minute until they release their aroma. The shrimp should be cooked for 2 to 3 minutes on all sides in the skillet until they reach a pink color. Take out the shrimp and put them to the side. As you pour the coconut milk and curry powder into the skillet, make sure to stir them thoroughly. Allow the flavors to combine by simmering for a period of 5 minutes. The lime juice should be stirred in, and then salt and pepper should be added. Put the shrimp back into the skillet and continue to cook for an additional 2 minutes. In an alternative skillet, sauté the cauliflower rice for 3 to 4 minutes, or until it reaches the desired tenderness. Present the shrimp coconut curry over the cauliflower rice, garnished with fresh cilantro.

Nutritional Info: Calories: 330 kcal, Protein: 25g, Carbohydrates: 15g, Fat: 20g, Saturated Fat: 15g, Cholesterol: 170mg, Sodium: 510mg, Potassium: 850mg, Sugars: 4g

8. Grilled Eggplant with Walnut Pesto and Arugula Salad

This Mediterranean-inspired dish is packed with anti-inflammatory ingredients such as eggplant, walnuts, and arugula. Eggplant is rich in fiber and antioxidants, while walnuts provide omega-3 fatty acids to support heart and brain health in women over 60.

(Ready in: 30 minutes | Cook Duration: 15 minutes | Persons: 2)

Necessary Items:

- Eggplant: 1 large, sliced into rounds
- Olive oil: 2 tbsps
- Walnuts: 1/4 cup, toasted
- Fresh basil: 1/2 cup, severed
- Garlic: 1 piece, crushed
- Lemon juice: 1 tbsp
- Arugula: 2 cups, fresh
- Parmesan (optional): 1 tbsp, grated
- Sea salt: 1/2 tsp
- Black pepper: 1/4 tsp

How to Prepare: Bring the temperature of your grill up to medium-high. Salt and pepper should be applied to the eggplant slices after they have been brushed with olive oil. When the eggplant is soft and has a small, charred appearance, grill it for 3 to 4 minutes on all sides. Put the walnuts, basil, garlic, lemon juice, and 1 tbsp of olive oil into a food processor and pulse until everything is combined. To make the pesto, pulse the ingredients until they are completely smooth. Take the leftover olive oil and toss it with the arugula. Season it with a little bit of salt and pepper. Present the grilled eggplant with a dollop of walnut pesto and the arugula salad on the side. Garnish with grated Parmesan if desired.

Nutritional Info: Calories: 280 kcal, Protein: 6g, Carbohydrates: 15g, Fat: 24g, Saturated Fat: 3g, Cholesterol: 0mg, Sodium: 290mg, Potassium: 750mg, Sugars: 5g

9. Quinoa and Roasted Vegetable Casserole with Almonds

This wholesome casserole combines quinoa and a mix of roasted vegetables, offering a hearty meal packed with fiber, antioxidants, and protein. Almonds add crunch and healthy fats, making it perfect for maintaining energy levels and supporting joint health in women over 60.

(Ready in: 45 minutes | Cook Duration: 35 minutes | Persons: 2)

Necessary Items:

- Quinoa: 1 cup, uncooked
- Mixed vegetables (including zucchini, bell peppers, and carrots): 3 cups, severed
- Olive oil: 2 tbsps
- Garlic: 2 pieces, crushed
- Almonds: 1/4 cup, severed
- Fresh thyme: 1 tbsp, severed
- Vegetable broth: 2 cups
- Sea salt: 1/2 tsp
- Black pepper: 1/4 tsp

How to Prepare: Warm up your oven to 375 deg.F (190 deg.C). Use 1 tbsp of olive oil, garlic, salt, and pepper to season the chopped vegetables, and then toss them together. Put them on a baking sheet and roast them for 20 to 25 minutes, or until they are soft.

While the veggies are roasting, prepare the quinoa in the vegetable broth corresponding to the directions on the package (this should take for around 15 minutes). After the quinoa has been allowed to cook and the veggies have been roasted, blend the two components in a baking dish. The topping should be topped with severed almonds and fresh thyme. Allow the dish to bake for 10 minutes so that the flavors can combine effectively. Present warm.

Nutritional Info: Calories: 400 kcal, Protein: 12g, Carbohydrates: 45g, Fat: 20g, Saturated Fat: 2.5g, Cholesterol: 0mg, Sodium: 320mg, Potassium: 950mg, Sugars: 8g

10. Grass-Fed Beef Stir-Fry with Ginger and Snap Peas

Grass-fed beef provides a lean source of protein with higher levels of omega-3 fatty acids than conventional beef. Paired with ginger and snap peas, this stir-fry is rich in anti-inflammatory compounds and antioxidants that support joint and heart health in women over 60.

(Prep Time: 25mins | Cook Time: 15 mins | Servings: 2)

Ingredients:

- Grass-fed beef strips: 8 oz
- Snap peas: 1 cup
- Red bell pepper: 1, sliced
- Fresh ginger: 1 tbsp, grated
- Garlic: 2 pieces, crushed
- Soy sauce (or tamari for gluten-free): 2 tbsps
- Sesame oil: 1 tbsp
- Olive oil: 1 tbsp
- Green onions: 2, severed
- Black pepper: 1/4 tsp

Instructions: In a big skillet or wok, bring the olive oil to a temp. on the medium-high side. After adding the beef strips, continue to cook them for 3 to 4 minutes until they have a browned appearance. The beef should be taken out and put away. While the sesame oil is heating up in the same skillet, sauté the garlic, ginger, snap peas, and bell pepper for 3 to 4 minutes, or until the vegetables are crisp-tender. The beef should be returned to the skillet, and the soy sauce and green onions should be stirred in. Continue to cook for a further 2 minutes while thoroughly combining the components. Present the stir-fry hot, garnished with more green onions if desired.

Nutritional Info: Calories: 380 kcal, Protein: 30g, Carbohydrates: 15g, Fat: 22g, Saturated Fat: 6g, Cholesterol: 70mg, Sodium: 590mg, Potassium: 650mg, Sugars: 4g

11. Spaghetti Squash with Tomato Basil Sauce and Turkey Meatballs

This light and flavorful dish replaces traditional pasta with spaghetti squash, a low-carb and fiber-rich vegetable. Paired with lean turkey meatballs and a fresh tomato basil sauce, it's a nutritious meal that supports heart and digestive health for women over 60.

(Ready in: 50 minutes | Cook Duration: 40 minutes | Persons: 2)

Necessary Items:

- Spaghetti squash: 1 medium
- Ground turkey: 8 oz
- Egg: 1
- Almond flour: 1/4 cup
- Garlic: 2 pieces, crushed
- Fresh basil: 2 tbsps, severed
- Crushed tomatoes (canned): 1 cup
- Olive oil: 2 tbsps
- Sea salt: 1/2 tsp
- Black pepper: 1/4 tsp
- Parmesan (optional): 1 tbsp, grated for garnish

How to Prepare: Warm up your oven to 375 deg.F (190 deg.C). You should first scoop out the seeds from the spaghetti squash, then cut it in half lengthwise, and then drizzle it with 1 tbsp of olive oil. Use pepper and salt to season the food. To achieve tenderness, roast for 35 to 40 minutes. During the time that the squash is roasting, mix together in a bowl the ground turkey, the egg, the almond flour, half of the garlic, salt, and pepper. Form into meatballs of a little size. In a skillet, warm 1 tbsp of olive oil and cook the meatballs for 6 to 8 minutes, turning them over to ensure that they are browned on both sides. Prepare the smashed tomatoes, the rest of the garlic, and the basil by heating them in a saucepan. While the mixture is simmering for ten minutes, flavor it to taste with salt and pepper. Using a fork, scrape the flesh of the squash into strands that resemble spaghetti once the squash is done cooking. While the spaghetti squash is being served, serve the turkey meatballs, topped with tomato sauce and optional Parmesan.

Nutritional Info: Calories: 370 kcal, Protein: 28g, Carbohydrates: 22g, Fat: 18g, Saturated Fat: 4g, Cholesterol: 110mg, Sodium: 520mg, Potassium: 960mg, Sugars: 9g

12. Vegan Chili with Sweet Potatoes and Avocado

This hearty vegan chili features sweet potatoes, black beans, and avocado, offering a rich source of fiber, plant-based protein, and healthy fats. It's perfect for promoting inflammation reduction and providing sustained energy for women over 60.

(Ready in: 40 minutes | Cook Duration: 30 minutes | Persons: 2)

Necessary Items:

- Sweet potato: 1 large, skinned and cubed
- Black beans (canned): 1 cup, drained and rinsed
- Diced tomatoes (canned): 1 cup
- Onion: 1 small, cubed
- Garlic: 2 pieces, crushed
- Chili powder: 1 tbsp
- Cumin: 1 tsp
- Olive oil: 1 tbsp
- Avocado: 1, cubed
- Fresh cilantro: 2 tbsps, severed
- Sea salt: 1/2 tsp
- Black pepper: 1/4 tsp

How to Prepare: In a big saucepan, bring the olive oil to a middling temp. Sauté the onion and garlic for 3 to 4 minutes, or until they have become more pliable. Sweet potato, chili powder, cumin, salt, and pepper should be added to the mixture. Coat the potatoes with the spices by stirring them thoroughly. Diced tomatoes and black beans should be added to the mixture.

Cook the chili for 20 to 25 minutes, or until the sweet potatoes are cooked, after bringing it to a simmer. Present the chili in bowls, topped with cubed avocado and fresh cilantro.

Nutritional Info: Calories: 360 kcal, Protein: 9g, Carbohydrates: 50g, Fat: 14g, Saturated Fat: 2g, Cholesterol: 0mg, Sodium: 470mg, Potassium: 1050mg, Sugars: 12g

13. Broiled Mackerel with Citrus Slaw and Roasted Brussels Sprouts

Mackerel is an omega-3 rich fish that supports heart and brain health, making it a great choice for an anti-inflammatory dinner. Paired with a refreshing citrus slaw and fiber-rich Brussels sprouts, this dish is ideal for women over 60.

(Prep Time: 35 minutes | Cook Time: 25 minutes | Servings: 2)

Ingredients:

- Mackerel fillets: 2 (4 oz each)
- Brussels sprouts: 2 cups, halved
- Olive oil: 2 tbsps
- Orange juice: 2 tbsps
- Red cabbage: 1 cup, shredded
- Carrot: 1 small, grated
- Apple cider vinegar: 1 tbsp
- Dijon mustard: 1 tsp
- Sea salt: 1/2 tsp
- Black pepper: 1/4 tsp

Instructions: Warm up your oven to 400 deg.F (200 deg.C). Brussels sprouts should be tossed with 1 tbsp of olive oil, salt, and pepper before being served. To achieve a crispy texture, roast for 20 to 25 minutes. During the time that the Brussels sprouts are roasting, mix together in a bowl the red cabbage, carrot, orange juice, apple cider vinegar, Dijon mustard, and a little bit of salt. Put away for later. Put the oven on broiler mode. Mackerel fillets should be placed on a baking pan, drizzled with 1 tbsp of olive oil, and seasoned with salt and pepper before being placed in the oven. Broil the fish for 5 to 7 minutes, or until it is golden brown and cooked all the way through. Present the broiled mackerel with the citrus slaw and roasted Brussels sprouts on the side.

Nutritional Info: Calories: 400 kcal, Protein: 28g, Carbohydrates: 22g, Fat: 24g, Saturated Fat: 4g, Cholesterol: 85mg, Sodium: 410mg, Potassium: 900mg, Sugars: 10g

14. Seared Tuna Steak with Avocado Salad and Lime Dressing

This quick and nutritious dish features tuna, a lean source of protein and omega-3s, paired with a vibrant avocado salad. The lime dressing adds a refreshing tang, making it perfect for promoting heart health and joint mobility in women over 60.

(Ready in: 20 minutes, Cook Duration: 10 minutes, Persons: 2)

Necessary Items:

- Tuna steaks: 2 (4 oz each)
- Avocado: 1, cubed
- Cherry tomatoes: 1/2 cup, halved
- Red onion: 1/4 cup, cubed
- Lime: 1, juiced
- Olive oil: 2 tbsps

- Fresh cilantro: 1 tbsp, severed
- Black pepper: 1/4 tsp
- Sea salt: 1/2 tsp

How to Prepare: The olive oil, which is 1 tbsp, should be heated in a skillet at high temp. Once the tuna steaks have been seasoned with salt and pepper, sear them for 2 to 3 minutes on all sides for medium-rare, or cook them until they reach the level of doneness that you choose. Diced avocado, cherry tomatoes, red onion, lime juice, cilantro, and the rest of the olive oil should be mixed together in a bowl. After giving it a light toss, season it with salt and pepper. Present the seared tuna with the avocado salad on the side.

Nutritional Info: Calories: 320 kcal, Protein: 28g, Carbohydrates: 10g, Fat: 20g, Saturated Fat: 3g, Cholesterol: 50mg, Sodium: 390mg, Potassium: 800mg, Sugars: 3g

15. Mediterranean Stuffed Eggplant with Feta and Pine Nuts

This Mediterranean-inspired dish is packed with fiber, healthy fats, and antioxidants from the eggplant, feta, and pine nuts. It's an excellent meal to support heart health, joint flexibility, and balanced digestion in women over 60.

(Prep Time: 50 minutes, Cook Time: 40 minutes, Servings: 2)

Ingredients:

- Eggplant: 1 big, halved
- Garlic: 2 pieces, crushed
- Feta cheese: 1/4 cup, crumbled
- Olive oil: 2 tbsps
- Pine nuts: 2 tbsps, toasted
- Fresh parsley: 2 tbsps, severed
- Cherry tomatoes: 1/2 cup, halved
- Sea salt: 1/2 tsp
- Red onion: 1/4 cup, cubed
- Black pepper: 1/4 tsp

Instructions: Warm up your oven to 375 deg.F (190 deg.C). The meat of the eggplant should be removed with a spoon, leaving a border of approximately one-quarter of an inch around the skin. Remove the flesh from the eggplant and set it aside. Prepare 1 tbsp of olive oil by heating it in a skillet. Garlic, red onion, and sliced eggplant flesh should be sautéed for 5 to 7 minutes, or until the eggplant flesh has become more tender. The cherry tomatoes, half of the parsley, salt, and pepper should be stirred in at this point. Keep cooking for an additional 2 minutes. The eggplant halves should be filled with the vegetable mixture, and then feta cheese and pine nuts should be sprinkled on top. Include the rest of the olive oil, then bake the eggplant for 25 to 30 minutes, or until it reaches the desired tenderness.

Nutritional Info: Calories: 350 kcal, Protein: 10g, Carbohydrates: 25g, Fat: 25g, Saturated Fat: 6g, Cholesterol: 25mg, Sodium: 540mg, Potassium: 750mg, Sugars: 10g

16. Baked Turkey Meatloaf with Mashed Cauliflower

This lighter version of a traditional meatloaf is made with lean ground turkey and served with creamy mashed cauliflower, offering high protein and low-carb content. It's perfect for women over 60, supporting muscle health and balanced blood sugar levels.

(Ready in: 55 minutes | Cook Duration: 45 minutes | Persons: 2)

Necessary Items:

- Ground turkey: 12 oz
- Egg: 1
- Almond flour: 1/4 cup
- Onion: 1 small, cubed
- Garlic: 2 pieces, crushed
- Tomato paste: 2 tbsps
- Worcestershire sauce: 1 tbsp
- Fresh parsley: 2 tbsps, severed
- Cauliflower: 1 head, severed into florets
- Olive oil: 2 tbsps
- Sea salt: 1/2 tsp
- Black pepper: 1/4 tsp

How to Prepare: Warm up the oven to 375 deg.F (190 deg.C). The ground turkey, egg, almond flour, onion, garlic, tomato paste, Worcestershire sauce, parsley, salt, and pepper should be mixed together in a bowl. Create a loaf out of the batter, and then set it in a baking dish that has been oiled. Bake for 40 to 45 minutes, or until the food is completely done. In the meantime, steam the cauliflower florets for 8 to 10 minutes, or until they are tender. Blend the cauliflower that has been steamed with olive oil, salt, and pepper until it is completely smooth. Present the sliced turkey meatloaf with a side of mashed cauliflower.

Nutritional Info: Calories: 420 kcal, Protein: 35g, Carbohydrates: 18g, Fat: 22g, Saturated Fat: 5g, Cholesterol: 140mg, Sodium: 670mg, Potassium: 900mg, Sugars: 7g

17. Roasted Brussels Sprouts with Almond-Crusted Salmon

This nourishing dish features omega-3 rich salmon, crusted with almonds for extra crunch and healthy fats. Paired with roasted Brussels sprouts, it's an excellent choice for supporting joint health and reducing inflammation in women over 60.

(Ready in: 35 minutes | Cook Duration: 25 minutes | Persons: 2)

Necessary Items:

- Salmon fillets: 2 (4 oz each)
- Almonds: 1/4 cup, finely severed
- Dijon mustard: 1 tbsp
- Brussels sprouts: 2 cups, halved
- Olive oil: 2 tbsps
- Sea salt: 1/2 tsp
- Black pepper: 1/4 tsp
- Lemon: 1/2, for garnish

How to Prepare: Warm up the oven to 400 deg.F (200 deg.C). Brussels sprouts should be tossed with 1 tbsp of olive oil, salt, and pepper before being served. To achieve a crispy texture, roast for 20 to 25 minutes. While this is going on, coat the salmon fillets with Dijon mustard and then press the severed almonds onto the top of each fillet. Put the salmon on a baking sheet that has been prepared with parchment paper and bake it for 12 to 15 minutes, or until the fish is fully cooked and the almonds have turned a golden color. Present the almond-crusted salmon with roasted Brussels sprouts and a wedge of lemon.

Nutritional Info: Calories: 450 kcal, Protein: 30g, Carbohydrates: 18g, Fat: 30g, Saturated Fat: 4g, Cholesterol: 65mg, Sodium: 420mg, Potassium: 850mg, Sugars: 6g

18. Grilled Lamb Chops with Minted Quinoa Salad

Lamb chops provide a rich source of protein and iron, supporting muscle and energy levels. Paired with a refreshing minted quinoa salad, this dish is ideal for promoting heart health and reducing inflammation in women over 60.

(Ready in: 30 minutes | Cook Duration: 15 minutes | Persons: 2)

Necessary Items:

- Lamb chops: 4 small
- Olive oil: 2 tbsps
- Garlic: 2 pieces, crushed
- Fresh mint: 2 tbsps, severed
- Quinoa: 1/2 cup
- Cucumber: 1/2, cubed
- Cherry tomatoes: 1/2 cup, halved
- Lemon juice: 1 tbsp
- Sea salt: 1/2 tsp
- Black pepper: 1/4 tsp

How to Prepare: Prepare the quinoa in accordance with the directions provided on the package, and then put it away to gently cool. Put the garlic, salt, pepper, and olive oil into a small bowl and mix them together. The lamb chops should be rubbed with the mixture. Cook the lamb chops for 3 to 4 minutes on all sides, or until they reach the desired level of doneness, on a grill or grill pan that has been heated at med-high temp. Toss the quinoa with cucumber, cherry tomatoes, mint, and lemon juice. Present alongside the grilled lamb chops.

Nutritional Info: Calories: 510 kcal, Protein: 35g, Carbohydrates: 30g, Fat: 28g, Saturated Fat: 10g, Cholesterol: 90mg, Sodium: 380mg, Potassium: 720mg, Sugars: 5g

19. Quinoa Risotto with Mushrooms and Spinach

This creamy quinoa risotto provides a gluten-free alternative to traditional risotto, while delivering plant-based protein and fiber. It's a delicious option for reducing inflammation and promoting digestive health for women over 60.

(Ready in: 35 minutes | Cook Duration: 30 minutes | Persons: 2)

Ingredients:

- Quinoa: 1/2 cup
- Mushrooms: 1 cup, sliced
- Spinach: 2 cups
- Onion: 1 small, cubed
- Garlic: 2 pieces, crushed
- Vegetable broth: 2 cups
- Olive oil: 2 tbsps
- Nutritional yeast: 2 tbsps (optional, for added flavor)
- Sea salt: 1/2 tsp
- Black pepper: 1/4 tsp

Instructions: The onion and garlic should be sautéed in a big skillet with 1 tbsp of olive oil for 2 to 3 minutes, or until they have become more tender. Cook the mushrooms for a further 5 minutes after adding them. It is then brought to a simmer once the quinoa and vegetable broth have been stirred in.

Cook the quinoa for 15 to 20 minutes, or until it is soft and the majority of the liquid has been absorbed. Once the spinach has been wilted, stir it in and continue cooking for an additional 2 minutes. Add nutritional yeast (if using), salt, and pepper.

Nutritional Info: Calories: 360 kcal, Protein: 14g, Carbohydrates: 50g, Fat: 12g, Saturated Fat: 2g, Cholesterol: 0mg, Sodium: 480mg, Potassium: 900mg, Sugars: 8g

20. Coconut-Braised Tempeh with Bok Choy and Carrots

This vegan-friendly dish combines protein-rich tempeh with nutrient-dense bok choy and carrots, all braised in coconut milk. It's perfect for women, supporting bone and heart health.

(Ready in: 30 minutes, Cook Duration: 20mins, Persons: 2)

Necessary Items:

- Tempeh: 1 block (8 oz), sliced
- Bok choy: 2 heads, severed
- Carrots: 2, sliced
- Coconut milk (light): 1 cup
- Soy sauce (low-sodium): 1 tbsp
- Ginger: 1-inch piece, grated
- Garlic: 2 pieces, crushed
- Olive oil: 1 tbsp
- Sea salt: 1/2 tsp
- Black pepper: 1/4 tsp

How to Prepare: In a big skillet, bring the olive oil to a middling temp. The tempeh slices should be cooked for 3 to 4 minutes on all sides until they reach a golden brown color. Get rid of the tempeh and put it to the side. Put the garlic, ginger, carrots, and bok choy in the same skillet as the other components. Sauté for a period of 5 minutes. It is important to whisk the coconut milk and soy sauce together after pouring them in. Put the vegetables on a low simmer for 10 minutes, or until they are soft. Repeat the process of adding the tempeh to the skillet and continuing to cook it for an additional 2 to 3 minutes. Use pepper and salt to season the food. Present the coconut-braised tempeh with bok choy and carrots.

Nutritional Info: Calories: 420 kcal, Protein: 21g, Carbohydrates: 28g, Fat: 26g, Saturated Fat: 12g, Cholesterol: 0mg, Sodium: 580mg, Potassium: 750mg, Sugars: 8g

Chapter 9: Anti-Inflammatory Snack & Dessert Recipes

1. Matcha and Coconut Chia Pudding

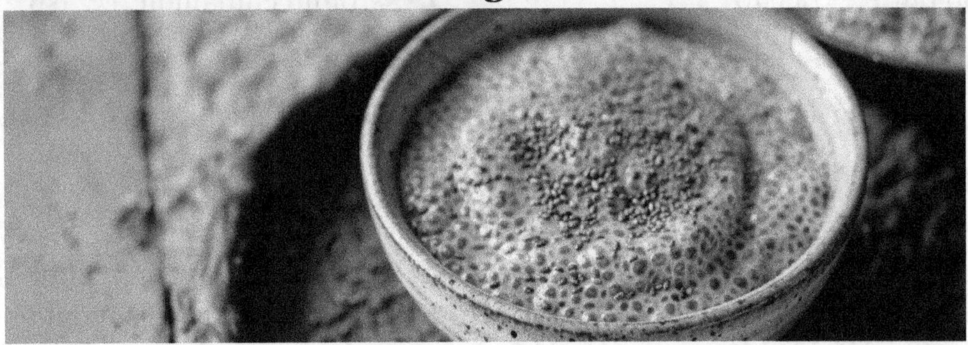

This refreshing Matcha and Coconut Chia Pudding is rich in antioxidants and healthy fats, making it a perfect anti-inflammatory snack or dessert for women over 60. Matcha helps to reduce inflammation while chia seeds provide fiber and omega-3s, which support heart and brain health.

(Ready in: 10 minutes | Chill Duration: 2 hours | Servings: 2)

Necessary Items:

- Chia seeds: 1/4 cup
- Unsweetened coconut milk: 1 cup
- Matcha powder: 1 tsp
- Vanilla extract: 1/2 tsp
- Maple syrup or honey (optional, for sweetness): 1 tbsp
- Unsweetened shredded coconut (for topping): 2 tbsps
- Fresh berries (optional, for garnish): 1/4 cup

How to Prepare: To ensure that the coconut milk, matcha powder, vanilla extract, and maple syrup (if using) are thoroughly mixed together, put them in a bowl and whisk them together. The chia seeds should be added and thoroughly mixed in. After allowing the mixture to sit for around 5 minutes, whisk it once more to avoid the chia seeds from clumping together. Make sure the bowl is covered and placed in the refrigerator for almost 2 hours or overnight. This will allow the chia seeds to absorb the liquid and develop a consistency similar to that of custard. When you are ready to serve the pudding, split it halfway between two bowls and, if you so wish, garnish each bowl with shredded coconut and fresh berries.

Nutritional Info: Calories: 170 kcal, Protein: 4g, Carbohydrates: 13g, Fat: 10g, Saturated Fat: 8g, Fiber: 8g, Sugar: 2g, Omega-3: 3g

2. Turmeric and Ginger Energy Balls

Turmeric and ginger are two potent anti-inflammatory ingredients that help reduce joint pain and stiffness, which are common concerns for women over 60. These energy balls are packed with healthy fats, fiber, and protein, making them a great option for a quick snack that supports an anti-inflammatory lifestyle.

(Ready in: 10 minutes | Chill Duration: 30 minutes | Servings: 10 balls)

Necessary Items:

- Rolled oats: 1/2 cup
- Almond butter: 1/4 cup
- Ground turmeric: 1 tsp
- Fresh grated ginger: 1 tsp
- Honey or maple syrup: 2 tbsps
- Chia seeds: 1 tbsp
- Ground cinnamon: 1/2 tsp
- Ground flaxseeds: 1 tbsp
- Unsweetened shredded coconut (for rolling): 1/4 cup

How to Prepare: Blend the oats, almond butter, turmeric, grated ginger, honey, chia seeds, ground cinnamon, and flaxseeds in a big bowl and stir them together until they are well incorporated. The mixture should be rolled into little balls, each of which should be around the size of a tbsp. Use shredded coconut to uniformly cover the energy balls by rolling them in the coconut. In order to ensure that the energy balls are firm before they are served, place them in the fridge for a minimum of 30 minutes.

Nutritional Info: Calories: 90 kcal, Protein: 2g, Carbohydrates: 9g, Fat: 5g, Fiber: 2g, Sugar: 4g, Omega-3: 1g

---

3. Baked Apple Slices with Cinnamon and Walnuts

This warm and comforting snack is rich in fiber and antioxidants. Apples contain pectin, a type of soluble fiber that can support gut health, while walnuts add healthy fats and help reduce inflammation, particularly in women over 60.

(Ready in: 5 minutes | Cook Duration: 25 minutes | Servings: 2)

Ingredients:

- Apples (such as Honeycrisp or Granny Smith): 2, finely cut
- Ground cinnamon: 1 tsp
- Walnuts: 1/4 cup, severed
- Maple syrup or honey: 1 tbsp (optional)
- Coconut oil: 1 tsp

Instructions: Warm up the oven to 175 deg.C (350 deg.F). Put the apple slices on a baking sheet that has been lined with parchment paper and organize them in a single layer. Drizzle the apple pieces with melted coconut oil and sprinkle with cinnamon. Add severed walnuts evenly across the apple pieces, and drizzle with maple syrup or honey if you prefer extra sweetness. Bake the apples for 20 to 25 minutes, or until they are golden and soft. Present when still heated.

Nutritional Info: Calories: 160 kcal, Protein: 2g, Carbohydrates: 23g, Fat: 8g, Fiber: 4g, Sugar: 15g, Omega-3: 0.8g

4. Dark Chocolate-Dipped Strawberries with Pistachios

This antioxidant-rich snack combines the benefits of dark chocolate and strawberries. Dark chocolate is packed with anti-inflammatory flavonoids, while strawberries offer vitamins and antioxidants that promote heart health, especially important for women over 60. The added crunch of pistachios brings healthy fats and fiber, making this a guilt-free treat.

(Ready in: 10 minutes | Chill Duration: 10 minutes | Servings: 4)

Ingredients:

- Fresh strawberries: 12 large

- Dark chocolate (70% cocoa or higher): 3 oz, melted

- Shelled pistachios: 1/4 cup, finely severed

Instructions: Perform a thorough washing and drying of the strawberries. In a bowl that is safe for use in the microwave, melt the dark chocolate by heating it in increments of 30 seconds and stirring it between all of them until it is completely melted and smooth. Each strawberry should be dipped into the melted dark chocolate, and any extra should be allowed to drip off. Sprinkle the severed pistachios onto the chocolate-dipped strawberries. Place the strawberries on a parchment-lined tray and refrigerate for 10 minutes, or until the chocolate has hardened. Present chilled.

Nutritional Info: Calories: 120 kcal, Protein: 2g, Carbohydrates: 14g, Fat: 8g, Fiber: 3g, Sugar: 8g, Omega-3: 0.1g

5. Almond Butter Stuffed Dates with Hemp Seeds

Almond Butter Stuffed Dates are a nutrient-packed snack that satisfies sweet cravings while supporting inflammation reduction. Dates provide natural sweetness and fiber, while almond butter delivers healthy fats and protein. Hemp seeds, rich in omega-3 fatty acids, further boost the anti-inflammatory benefits, making this an ideal snack for women over 60.

(Ready in: 5 minutes | Servings: 6)

Necessary Items:

- Medjool dates: 6, pitted

- Almond butter: 2 tbsps

- Hemp seeds: 1 tbsp

How to Prepare: Slice each date lengthwise to create an opening, but don't cut all the way through. Spoon about half a tsp of almond butter into the center of each date. Sprinkle the stuffed dates with hemp seeds for added texture and omega-3 goodness. You can present it right away, or you can put it in the refrigerator to keep it chilled.

Nutritional Info: Calories: 120 kcal, Protein: 2g, Carbohydrates: 19g, Fat: 5g, Fiber: 3g, Sugar: 16g, Omega-3: 0.6g

6. Coconut Yogurt with Fresh Mango and Chia Seeds

This refreshing snack is loaded with healthy fats, fiber, and vitamins. Coconut yogurt offers dairy-free probiotics that support gut health, while mango provides a burst of vitamin C and antioxidants. Chia seeds are rich in omega-3s, which help reduce inflammation—making this the perfect anti-inflammatory snack for women over 60.

(Ready in: 5 minutes | Servings: 2)

Necessary Items:

- Coconut yogurt: 1 cup

- Fresh mango: 1/2 cup, cubed

- Chia seeds: 1 tbsp

How to Prepare: Spoon the coconut yogurt into two serving bowls. Top each bowl with cubed mango. Chia seeds, which are rich in omega-3 fatty acids and fiber, should be sprinkled over the mango and yoghurt.

Nutritional Info: Calories: 180 kcal, Protein: 3g, Carbohydrates: 25g, Fat: 7g, Fiber: 6g, Sugar: 16g, Omega-3: 1.8g

7. Flaxseed Crackers with Hummus

Flaxseed crackers are a crunchy, fiber-packed snack rich in omega-3 fatty acids, which help reduce inflammation. Paired with protein-rich hummus, this combination supports healthy digestion and sustained energy.

(Ready in: 10 minutes | Servings: 2)

Necessary Items:

- Flaxseed crackers: 6

- Hummus: 1/4 cup

How to Prepare: Arrange flaxseed crackers on a serving plate. Scoop the hummus into a small bowl for dipping or spread directly onto the crackers. Enjoy as a quick and nutritious snack.

Nutritional Info: Calories: 150 kcal, Protein: 4g, Carbohydrates: 12g, Fat: 10g, Fiber: 7g, Sugar: 1g, Omega-3: 2.5g

8. Oat and Date Cookies with Cinnamon

These soft, naturally sweet cookies are made with oats and dates, which are both high in fiber and help promote digestive health. Cinnamon adds a touch of warmth and has anti-inflammatory properties, making these cookies a satisfying snack for women over 60 who need a sweet yet wholesome option.

(Ready in: 15 minutes | Bake Duration: 12 minutes | Servings: 8)

Necessary Items:

- Rolled oats: 1 cup

- Medjool dates: 6, pitted and severed

- Almond flour: 1/4 cup
- Coconut oil: 2 tbsps, melted
- Ground cinnamon: 1 tsp
- Vanilla extract: 1/2 tsp

How to Prepare. Line a baking sheet with parchment paper and preheat the oven to 175 deg.C (350 deg.F). In a bowl, mix together the oats, dates that have been diced, almond flour, and cinnamon. After thoroughly combining the dry components, add the melted coconut oil and vanilla essence and stir until everything is incorporated. Prepare the dough by rolling it into little balls and then flattening them into cookie shapes on the baking sheet. To achieve a golden-brown color, bake for 10 to 12 minutes. Prior to presenting, allow to cool.

Nutritional Info: Calories: 110 kcal, Protein: 2g, Carbohydrates: 18g, Fat: 5g, Fiber: 3g, Sugar: 7g, Omega-3: 0.1g

---

9. Roasted Chickpeas with Paprika and Turmeric

Roasted chickpeas make a crunchy, savory snack packed with plant-based protein and fiber. The paprika and turmeric add anti-inflammatory benefits while giving these chickpeas a warm, slightly spicy flavor. This snack is ideal for women over 60 seeking a heart-healthy, flavorful option.

(Ready in: 10 minutes | Roast Duration: 25 minutes | Servings: 4)

Necessary Items:

- Canned chickpeas: 1 can (15 oz), drained and rinsed
- Olive oil: 1 tbsp
- Paprika: 1/2 tsp
- Turmeric: 1/2 tsp
- Salt: as required

How to Prepare: Arrange a baking sheet with parchment paper and warm up the oven to 400 deg.F (200 deg.C). After drying them with a paper towel, the chickpeas should be spread out on the baking sheet and put into the oven. Salt, paprika, and turmeric should be sprinkled on top after the olive oil has been drizzled over. To ensure a uniform coating, toss the components. Roast the chickpeas for 25 to 30 minutes, stirring the pan halfway through the cooking process, until they are golden and crispy. Let cool slightly before serving.

Nutritional Info: Calories: 130 kcal, Protein: 6g, Carbohydrates: 19g, Fat: 4g, Fiber: 5g, Sugar: 1g, Omega-3: 0.1g

---

10. Turmeric-Spiced Cashew Nuts

Cashews are a great source of healthy fats and magnesium, which support bone health in women over 60. Turmeric adds a powerful anti-inflammatory boost to this simple snack, making it both delicious and beneficial for overall wellness.

(Ready in: 5 minutes | Toast Duration: 5 minutes | Servings: 4)

Ingredients:

- Raw cashew nuts: 1 cup
- Olive oil: 1 tbsp
- Ground turmeric: 1/2 tsp
- Sea salt: as required

Instructions: Warm a skillet at middling temp. and include the olive oil. Stir in the cashews and sprinkle with turmeric and sea salt. Toast the cashews for 5-7 minutes, stirring frequently, until golden and fragrant. Let cool before serving as a crunchy, nutrient-packed snack.

Nutritional Info: Calories: 180 kcal, Protein: 5g, Carbohydrates: 9g, Fat: 14g, Fiber: 1g, Sugar: 2g, Omega-3: 0.2g

11. Pumpkin Seed and Dark Chocolate Bark

Pumpkin seeds are rich in magnesium, which supports bone health, while dark chocolate provides powerful antioxidants that help reduce inflammation. This easy-to-make bark is a crunchy, satisfying treat for women over 60, combining healthy fats with a touch of sweetness.

(Ready in: 10 minutes | Chill Duration: 20 minutes | Servings: 6)

Necessary Items:

- Dark chocolate (70% cocoa or higher): 1 cup, melted

- Pumpkin seeds: 1/4 cup, toasted

- Sea salt: pinch

How to Prepare: Put parchment paper in a baking pan and put it away. The dark chocolate that has been melted should be poured onto the sheet, and then it should be spread out in a uniform layer. To finish off the chocolate, sprinkle some toasted pumpkin seeds and a little bit of sea salt on top. Place the sheet in the fridge for 20 minutes or until the chocolate hardens. Break the bark into pieces and enjoy.

Nutritional Info: Calories: 180 kcal, Protein: 3g, Carbohydrates: 18g, Fat: 13g, Fiber: 4g, Sugar: 9g, Omega-3: 0.1g

12. Apple and Almond Butter Sandwiches

These apple and almond butter sandwiches are a perfect combination of fiber and healthy fats. Apples provide important vitamins and antioxidants, while almond butter is rich in vitamin E, supporting skin health and inflammation reduction, making this an ideal snack for women over 60.

(Ready in: 5 minutes | Servings: 2)

Necessary Items:

- Apple: 1, sliced into rounds

- Almond butter: 2 tbsps

- Chia seeds: 1 tsp (optional)

How to Prepare: Slice the apple into thick, round pieces. Spread almond butter on half of the apple pieces. Sprinkle chia seeds on top of the almond butter for an extra fiber boost, if desired. Top each with the remaining apple pieces to form mini sandwiches.

Nutritional Info: Calories: 190 kcal, Protein: 4g, Carbohydrates: 24g, Fat: 9g, Fiber: 5g, Sugar: 16g, Omega-3: 0.4g

13. Ginger-Spiced Carrot Muffins

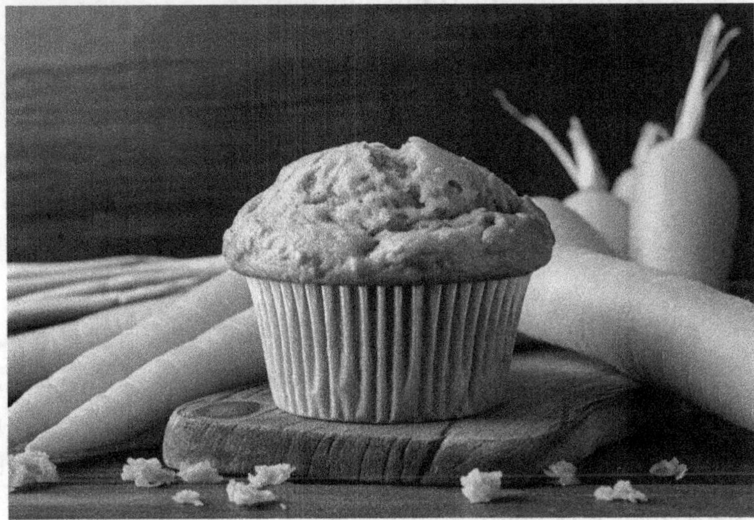

These moist, flavorful muffins are made with carrots, which are high in beta-carotene, and ginger, which has powerful anti-inflammatory properties. The combination of warming spices makes these muffins an excellent choice for women over 60 looking for a healthy, nutrient-packed snack.

(Ready in: 10 minutes | Bake Duration: 20 minutes | Servings: 8)

Ingredients:

- Whole wheat flour: 1 cup
- Grated carrots: 1 cup
- Ground ginger: 1 tsp
- Cinnamon: 1/2 tsp
- Baking powder: 1 tsp
- Coconut oil: 1/4 cup, melted
- Maple syrup: 1/4 cup
- Egg: 1

Instructions: Warm up the oven to 350 deg.F (175 deg.C), and line a muffin tray with paper liners. Put the flour, ginger, cinnamon, and baking powder into a bowl and mix them together. Coconut oil, maple syrup, and the egg should be mixed together in a separate basin using a whisk. To include the grated carrots, first stir the wet components into the dry mixture in an orderly manner until they are almost completely incorporated. The batter should be poured into the muffin tray, and the muffins should be baked for 18 to 20 minutes, or until a toothpick tests clean. Prior to presenting, allow to cool.

Nutritional Info: Calories: 160 kcal, Protein: 3g, Carbohydrates: 22g, Fat: 7g, Fiber: 3g, Sugar: 10g, Omega-3: 0.1g

14. Mixed Berry and Chia Seed Parfait

This vibrant parfait combines antioxidant-rich berries with omega-3-packed chia seeds, which help reduce inflammation and support heart health. It's an easy, nutritious snack perfect for women over 60 who want a refreshing, nutrient-dense treat.

(Ready in: 5 minutes | Servings: 2)

Ingredients:

- Greek yogurt (or coconut yogurt for dairy-free): 1 cup
- Mixed berries (blueberries, raspberries, strawberries): 1/2 cup
- Chia seeds: 1 tbsp
- Honey or maple syrup (optional): 1 tsp

Instructions: Layer half of the yogurt into two serving glasses. Top with mixed berries and sprinkle chia seeds over them. Add another layer of yogurt and finish with more berries on top. Present instantly after drizzling honey or maple syrup, if preferred, through the dish.

Nutritional Info: Calories: 150 kcal, Protein: 8g, Carbohydrates: 18g, Fat: 4g, Fiber: 5g, Sugar: 12g, Omega-3: 1.8g

15. Coconut Macaroons with Dark Chocolate Drizzle

These light and chewy coconut macaroons are naturally sweetened and gluten-free. Coconut provides healthy fats that support brain function, while dark chocolate adds antioxidants. This indulgent yet healthy dessert is perfect for women over 60 looking for a guilt-free treat.

(Ready in: 10 minutes | Bake Duration: 12 minutes | Servings: 8)

Necessary Items:

- Unsweetened shredded coconut: 1 cup
- Egg white: 1
- Maple syrup: 2 tbsps
- Vanilla extract: 1/2 tsp
- Dark chocolate (70% cocoa or higher): 1/4 cup, melted

How to Prepare: Line a baking sheet with parchment paper and warm up the oven to 175 deg.C (350 deg.F). Blend the shredded coconut, egg white, maple syrup, and vanilla essence in a bowl and stir until everything is incorporated. The mixture should be formed into small balls, which should then be placed on the baking sheet. Bake the macaroons for 10 to 12 minutes, or until they have a golden color. Once cooled, drizzle melted dark chocolate over the macaroons and allow the chocolate to set.

Nutritional Info: Calories: 120 kcal, Protein: 2g, Carbohydrates: 12g, Fat: 8g, Fiber: 3g, Sugar: 8g, Omega-3: 0.1g

16. Tahini and Honey Roasted Almonds

Almonds are a fantastic source of vitamin E and magnesium, both of which help reduce inflammation. Combined with tahini and honey, these roasted almonds offer a unique nutty-sweet flavor, making them a perfect snack for women over 60 looking to boost their heart health and energy levels.

(Ready in: 5 minutes | Cook Duration: 15 minutes | Servings: 6)

Necessary Items:

- Raw almonds: 1 cup

- Tahini: 2 tbsps

- Honey: 1 tbsp

- Sea salt: pinch

How to Prepare. Line a baking sheet with parchment paper and warm up the oven to 175 deg.C (350 deg.F). Honey and tahini should be combined in a bowl and made into a homogeneous paste. Following the addition of the almonds, toss them until they are equally covered. Place the almonds that have been coated in a single layer on the baking sheet that has been prepared. In a preheated oven, bake for 12 to 15 minutes, tossing halfway through, until thoroughly browned. Take the dish out of the oven, season it with salt from the sea, and allow it to cool prior to presenting.

Nutritional Info: Calories: 160 kcal, Protein: 5g, Carbohydrates: 10g, Fat: 12g, Fiber: 3g, Sugar: 5g, Omega-3: 0.1g

17. Peanut Butter and Coconut Balls

These no-bake peanut butter and coconut balls are a quick and easy snack packed with protein and healthy fats. Peanut butter offers a rich source of niacin and antioxidants, supporting brain function and heart health for women over 60, while coconut adds a touch of sweetness and fiber.

(Ready in: 10 minutes | Chill Duration: 20 minutes | Servings: 10)

Necessary Items:

- Peanut butter (natural, unsweetened): 1/2 cup

- Shredded coconut (unsweetened): 1/2 cup

- Honey: 2 tbsps

- Chia seeds: 1 tbsp

- Ground flaxseeds: 1 tbsp

How to Prepare. In a mixing bowl, blend peanut butter, shredded coconut, honey, chia seeds, and ground flaxseeds. Stir until the mixture is well combined. The mixture should be rolled into little balls with a diameter of approximately one inch. Put the balls in the fridge for 20 minutes so that they can toughen up. You can serve it right away, or you can put it in the fridge in a sealed container.

Nutritional Info: Calories: 110 kcal, Protein: 3g, Carbohydrates: 8g, Fat: 8g, Fiber: 2g, Sugar: 5g, Omega-3: 0.4g

18. Baked Sweet Potato Chips with Paprika

Sweet potatoes are rich in beta-carotene, which supports immune function and skin health. These crispy baked sweet potato chips seasoned with paprika make a delicious and healthy alternative to traditional chips, offering anti-inflammatory benefits for women over 60.

(Ready in: 10 minutes | Bake Duration: 25 minutes | Servings: 4)

Necessary Items:

- Sweet potatoes: 2 medium-sized
- Olive oil: 1 tbsp
- Paprika: 1 tsp
- Sea salt: pinch

How to Prepare. Using parchment paper, line a baking sheet and warm up the oven to 375 deg.F (190 deg.C). Cut the sweet potatoes into thin slices using a mandoline or a knife that is very sharp. The sweet potato slices should be tossed in a bowl with olive oil, paprika, and sea salt until they are equally covered with the seasonings. The slices should be spread out in a single layer on the baking sheet that has been prepared. Bake for 20 to 25 minutes, turning halfway through, until the food is golden brown and crispy. Prior to serving, allow it to mildly cool down.

Nutritional Info: Calories: 120 kcal, Protein: 2g, Carbohydrates: 20g, Fat: 4g, Fiber: 3g, Sugar: 5g, Omega-3: 0.1g

90-Day Anti-Inflammatory Meal Plan for Women Over 60

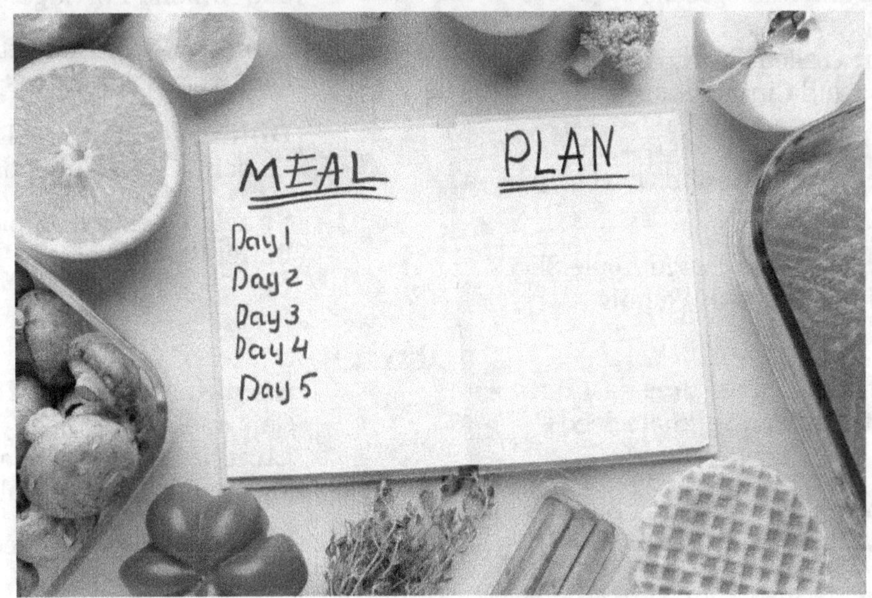

This 90-day anti-inflammatory meal plan is designed to support women over 60 in reducing inflammation, boosting energy, and enhancing well-being. Each meal in this plan is rich in antioxidants, healthy fats, and nutrient-dense ingredients that help combat inflammation and promote healthy aging. This plan includes breakfast, lunch, dinner, and snacks/desserts for every day, ensuring you enjoy a variety of meals that not only support your health but also delight your taste buds.

Day 1

Breakfast: Turmeric Oatmeal with Blueberries and Almonds

Lunch: Quinoa Salad with Avocado, Kale, and Pomegranate

Snack: Baked Salmon with Garlic and Rosemary Sweet Potatoes

Dinner: Matcha and Coconut Chia Pudding

Day 2

Breakfast: Chia Seed Pudding with Mixed Berries

Lunch: Chickpea and Spinach Stew with Coconut Milk

Dinner: Lentil and Vegetable Shepherd's Pie

Snack/Dessert: Turmeric and Ginger Energy Balls

Day 46

Breakfast: Buckwheat Pancakes with Fresh Raspberries

Lunch: Tuna Salad with Avocado and Cucumber on Mixed Greens

Dinner: Coconut-Curry Shrimp with Cauliflower Rice

Snack/Dessert: Turmeric-Spiced Cashew Nuts

Day 47

Breakfast: Anti-Inflammatory Green Smoothie with Kale and Pineapple

Lunch: Grilled Chicken Salad with Mixed Berries and Walnuts

Dinner: Grilled Eggplant with Walnut Pesto and Arugula Salad

Snack/Dessert: Pumpkin Seed and Dark Chocolate Bark

Day 3

Breakfast: Avocado Toast with Smoked Salmon and Microgreens

Lunch: Grilled Shrimp Salad with Arugula and Citrus Vinaigrette

Dinner: Turmeric and Ginger Chicken Stir-Fry with Broccoli

Snack/Dessert: Baked Apple Slices with Cinnamon and Walnuts

Day 4

Breakfast: Quinoa Breakfast Bowl with Walnuts and Pomegranate Seeds

Lunch: Sweet Potato and Black Bean Tacos with Avocado Salsa

Dinner: Grilled Tofu with Sesame Spinach and Brown Rice

Snack/Dessert: Dark Chocolate-Dipped Strawberries with Pistachios

Day 5

Breakfast: Greek Yogurt with Flaxseeds and Honey

Lunch: Cauliflower Rice Bowl with Tofu and Ginger-Sesame Dressing

Dinner: Wild-Caught Cod with Sautéed Spinach and Cherry Tomatoes

Snack/Dessert: Almond Butter Stuffed Dates with Hemp Seeds

Day 6

Breakfast: Buckwheat Pancakes with Fresh Raspberries

Lunch: Roasted Beet and Goat Cheese Salad with Walnuts

Dinner: Balsamic-Glazed Portobello Mushrooms with Zucchini Noodles

Snack/Dessert: Coconut Yogurt with Fresh Mango and Chia Seeds

Day 7

Breakfast: Anti-Inflammatory Green Smoothie with Kale and Pineapple

Lunch: Turmeric-Spiced Chicken Wrap

Day 48

Breakfast: Cinnamon-Spiced Apple and Almond Porridge

Lunch: Baked Cod with Herb-Infused Quinoa and Asparagus

Dinner: Quinoa and Roasted Vegetable Casserole with Almonds

Snack/Dessert: Apple and Almond Butter Sandwiches

Day 49

Breakfast: Coconut Yogurt Parfait with Chia and Hemp Seeds

Lunch: Sweet Potato and Black Bean Tacos with Avocado Salsa

Dinner: Grass-Fed Beef Stir-Fry with Ginger and Snap Peas

Snack/Dessert: Ginger-Spiced Carrot Muffins

Day 50

Breakfast: Flaxseed and Blueberry Smoothie Bowl

Lunch: Roasted Carrot and Parsnip Soup with Ginger

Dinner: Spaghetti Squash with Tomato Basil Sauce and Turkey Meatballs

Snack/Dessert: Mixed Berry and Chia Seed Parfait

Day 51

Breakfast: Almond Butter and Banana Rice Cakes

Lunch: Quinoa Salad with Avocado, Kale, and Pomegranate

Dinner: Vegan Chili with Sweet Potatoes and Avocado

Snack/Dessert: Coconut Macaroons with Dark Chocolate Drizzle

Day 52

Breakfast: Herb Omelet with Avocado and Arugula

Lunch: Chickpea and Spinach Stew

with Cucumber and Hummus

Dinner: Coconut-Curry Shrimp with Cauliflower Rice

Snack/Dessert: Flaxseed Crackers with Hummus

Day 8

Breakfast: Cinnamon-Spiced Apple and Almond Porridge

Lunch: Quinoa and Grilled Vegetable Buddha Bowl with Tahini Dressing

Dinner: Grilled Eggplant with Walnut Pesto and Arugula Salad

Snack/Dessert: Oat and Date Cookies with Cinnamon

Day 9

Breakfast: Coconut Yogurt Parfait with Chia and Hemp Seeds

Lunch: Tuna Salad with Avocado and Cucumber on Mixed Greens

Dinner: Quinoa and Roasted Vegetable Casserole with Almonds

Snack/Dessert: Roasted Chickpeas with Paprika and Turmeric

Day 10

Breakfast: Flaxseed and Blueberry Smoothie Bowl

Lunch: Chickpea and Cucumber Salad with Lemon-Tahini Dressing

Dinner: Grass-Fed Beef Stir-Fry with Ginger and Snap Peas

Snack/Dessert: Turmeric-Spiced Cashew Nuts

Day 11

Breakfast: Almond Butter and Banana Rice Cakes

Lunch: Baked Cod with Herb-Infused Quinoa and Asparagus

Dinner: Spaghetti Squash with Tomato Basil Sauce and Turkey Meatballs

Snack/Dessert: Pumpkin Seed and

with Coconut Milk

Dinner: Broiled Mackerel with Citrus Slaw and Roasted Brussels Sprouts

Snack/Dessert: Tahini and Honey Roasted Almonds

Day 53

Breakfast: Pumpkin and Ginger Smoothie

Lunch: Red Lentil and Sweet Potato Curry with Spinach

Dinner: Seared Tuna Steak with Avocado Salad and Lime Dressing

Snack/Dessert: Peanut Butter and Coconut Balls

Day 54

Breakfast: Zucchini and Carrot Breakfast Fritters

Lunch: Grilled Turkey Burgers with Avocado and Spinach

Dinner: Mediterranean Stuffed Eggplant with Feta and Pine Nuts

Snack/Dessert: Baked Sweet Potato Chips with Paprika

Day 55

Breakfast: Coconut Flour Waffles with Mixed Berries

Lunch: Spinach and Mushroom Frittata with Sweet Potatoes

Dinner: Baked Turkey Meatloaf with Mashed Cauliflower

Snack/Dessert: Matcha and Coconut Chia Pudding

Day 56

Breakfast: Matcha Smoothie with Spinach and Coconut Milk

Lunch: Grilled Salmon with Turmeric-Spiced Lentils

Dinner: Roasted Brussels Sprouts with Almond-Crusted Salmon

Snack/Dessert: Turmeric and Ginger

Dark Chocolate Bark

Energy Balls

Day 12

Breakfast: Herb Omelet with Avocado and Arugula

Lunch: Red Lentil and Sweet Potato Curry with Spinach

Dinner: Vegan Chili with Sweet Potatoes and Avocado

Snack/Dessert: Apple and Almond Butter Sandwiches

Day 13

Breakfast: Pumpkin and Ginger Smoothie

Lunch: Grilled Chicken Salad with Mixed Berries and Walnuts

Dinner: Broiled Mackerel with Citrus Slaw and Roasted Brussels Sprouts

Snack/Dessert: Ginger-Spiced Carrot Muffins

Day 14

Breakfast: Zucchini and Carrot Breakfast Fritters

Lunch: Roasted Carrot and Parsnip Soup with Ginger

Dinner: Seared Tuna Steak with Avocado Salad and Lime Dressing

Snack/Dessert: Mixed Berry and Chia Seed Parfait

Day 15

Breakfast: Coconut Flour Waffles with Mixed Berries

Lunch: Spinach and Mushroom Frittata with Sweet Potatoes

Dinner: Mediterranean Stuffed Eggplant with Feta and Pine Nuts

Snack/Dessert: Coconut Macaroons with Dark Chocolate Drizzle

Day 57

Breakfast: Poached Eggs with Avocado and Sautéed Greens

Lunch: Quinoa and Grilled Vegetable Buddha Bowl with Tahini Dressing

Dinner: Grilled Lamb Chops with Minted Quinoa Salad

Snack/Dessert: Baked Apple Slices with Cinnamon and Walnuts

Day 58

Breakfast: Cinnamon Quinoa with Almond Milk and Cherries

Lunch: Grilled Shrimp Salad with Arugula and Citrus Vinaigrette

Dinner: Quinoa Risotto with Mushrooms and Spinach

Snack/Dessert: Dark Chocolate-Dipped Strawberries with Pistachios

Day 59

Breakfast: Almond Flour Muffins with Turmeric and Ginger

Lunch: Sweet Potato and Black Bean Tacos with Avocado Salsa

Dinner: Coconut-Braised Tempeh with Bok Choy and Carrots

Snack/Dessert: Almond Butter Stuffed Dates with Hemp Seeds

Day 60

Breakfast: Anti-Inflammatory Smoothie with Mango, Turmeric, and Spinach

Lunch: Chickpea and Spinach Stew with Coconut Milk

Dinner: Baked Salmon with Garlic and Rosemary Sweet Potatoes

Snack/Dessert: Coconut Yogurt with Fresh Mango and Chia Seeds

Day 16

Breakfast: Matcha Smoothie with Spinach and Coconut Milk

Lunch: Black Bean and Quinoa Stuffed Zucchini Boats

Dinner: Baked Turkey Meatloaf with Mashed Cauliflower

Snack/Dessert: Tahini and Honey Roasted Almonds

Day 17

Breakfast: Poached Eggs with Avocado and Sautéed Greens

Lunch: Salmon Salad with Mixed Greens and Lemon-Tahini Dressing

Dinner: Roasted Brussels Sprouts with Almond-Crusted Salmon

Snack/Dessert: Peanut Butter and Coconut Balls

Day 18

Breakfast: Cinnamon Quinoa with Almond Milk and Cherries

Lunch: Roasted Chickpea and Avocado Wrap with Turmeric Hummus

Dinner: Grilled Lamb Chops with Minted Quinoa Salad

Snack/Dessert: Baked Sweet Potato Chips with Paprika

Day 19

Breakfast: Almond Flour Muffins with Turmeric and Ginger

Lunch: Cauliflower Rice Bowl with Tofu and Ginger-Sesame Dressing

Dinner: Quinoa Risotto with Mushrooms and Spinach

Snack/Dessert: Matcha and Coconut Chia Pudding

Day 20

Breakfast: Anti-Inflammatory Smoothie with Mango, Turmeric, and Spinach

Day 61

Breakfast: Turmeric Oatmeal with Blueberries and Almonds

Lunch: Grilled Turkey Burgers with Avocado and Spinach

Dinner: Wild-Caught Cod with Sautéed Spinach and Cherry Tomatoes

Snack/Dessert: Flaxseed Crackers with Hummus

Day 62

Breakfast: Chia Seed Pudding with Mixed Berries

Lunch: Quinoa Salad with Avocado, Kale, and Pomegranate

Dinner: Lentil and Vegetable Shepherd's Pie

Snack/Dessert: Oat and Date Cookies with Cinnamon

Day 63

Breakfast: Avocado Toast with Smoked Salmon and Microgreens

Lunch: Red Lentil and Sweet Potato Curry with Spinach

Dinner: Grass-Fed Beef Stir-Fry with Ginger and Snap Peas

Snack/Dessert: Roasted Chickpeas with Paprika and Turmeric

Day 64

Breakfast: Quinoa Breakfast Bowl with Walnuts and Pomegranate Seeds

Lunch: Roasted Beet and Goat Cheese Salad with Walnuts

Dinner: Grilled Eggplant with Walnut Pesto and Arugula Salad

Snack/Dessert: Turmeric-Spiced Cashew Nuts

Day 65

Breakfast: Greek Yogurt with Flaxseeds and Honey

Lunch: Chickpea and Cucumber Salad

Lunch: Grilled Turkey Burgers with Avocado and Spinach

Dinner: Coconut-Braised Tempeh with Bok Choy and Carrots

Snack/Dessert: Turmeric and Ginger Energy Balls

Day 21

Breakfast: Turmeric Oatmeal with Blueberries and Almonds

Lunch: Sweet Potato and Black Bean Tacos with Avocado Salsa

Dinner: Baked Salmon with Garlic and Rosemary Sweet Potatoes

Snack/Dessert: Baked Apple Slices with Cinnamon and Walnuts

Day 22

Breakfast: Chia Seed Pudding with Mixed Berries

Lunch: Chickpea and Spinach Stew with Coconut Milk

Dinner: Lentil and Vegetable Shepherd's Pie

Snack/Dessert: Dark Chocolate-Dipped Strawberries with Pistachios

Day 23

Breakfast: Avocado Toast with Smoked Salmon and Microgreens

Lunch: Quinoa Salad with Avocado, Kale, and Pomegranate

Dinner: Turmeric and Ginger Chicken Stir-Fry with Broccoli

Snack/Dessert: Almond Butter Stuffed Dates with Hemp Seeds

Day 24

Breakfast: Quinoa Breakfast Bowl with Walnuts and Pomegranate Seeds

Lunch: Grilled Shrimp Salad with Arugula and Citrus Vinaigrette

Dinner: Grilled Tofu with Sesame Spinach and Brown Rice

with Lemon-Tahini Dressing

Dinner: Spaghetti Squash with Tomato Basil Sauce and Turkey Meatballs

Snack/Dessert: Pumpkin Seed and Dark Chocolate Bark

Day 66

Breakfast: Buckwheat Pancakes with Fresh Raspberries

Lunch: Tuna Salad with Avocado and Cucumber on Mixed Greens

Dinner: Vegan Chili with Sweet Potatoes and Avocado

Snack/Dessert: Apple and Almond Butter Sandwiches

Day 67

Breakfast: Anti-Inflammatory Green Smoothie with Kale and Pineapple

Lunch: Grilled Chicken Salad with Mixed Berries and Walnuts

Dinner: Broiled Mackerel with Citrus Slaw and Roasted Brussels Sprouts

Snack/Dessert: Ginger-Spiced Carrot Muffins

Day 68

Breakfast: Cinnamon-Spiced Apple and Almond Porridge

Lunch: Baked Cod with Herb-Infused Quinoa and Asparagus

Dinner: Seared Tuna Steak with Avocado Salad and Lime Dressing

Snack/Dessert: Mixed Berry and Chia Seed Parfait

Day 69

Breakfast: Coconut Yogurt Parfait with Chia and Hemp Seeds

Lunch: Roasted Carrot and Parsnip Soup with Ginger

Dinner: Mediterranean Stuffed Eggplant with Feta and Pine Nuts

Snack/Dessert: Coconut Yogurt with Fresh Mango and Chia Seeds

Day 25

Breakfast: Greek Yogurt with Flaxseeds and Honey

Lunch: Sweet Potato and Black Bean Tacos with Avocado Salsa

Dinner: Wild-Caught Cod with Sautéed Spinach and Cherry Tomatoes

Snack/Dessert: Flaxseed Crackers with Hummus

Day 26

Breakfast: Buckwheat Pancakes with Fresh Raspberries

Lunch: Roasted Beet and Goat Cheese Salad with Walnuts

Dinner: Balsamic-Glazed Portobello Mushrooms with Zucchini Noodles

Snack/Dessert: Oat and Date Cookies with Cinnamon

Day 27

Breakfast: Anti-Inflammatory Green Smoothie with Kale and Pineapple

Lunch: Grilled Turkey Burgers with Avocado and Spinach

Dinner: Coconut-Curry Shrimp with Cauliflower Rice

Snack/Dessert: Roasted Chickpeas with Paprika and Turmeric

Day 28

Breakfast: Cinnamon-Spiced Apple and Almond Porridge

Lunch: Quinoa and Grilled Vegetable Buddha Bowl with Tahini Dressing

Dinner: Grilled Eggplant with Walnut Pesto and Arugula Salad

Snack/Dessert: Turmeric-Spiced Cashew Nuts

Day 29

Breakfast: Coconut Yogurt Parfait with Chia and Hemp Seeds

Snack/Dessert: Coconut Macaroons with Dark Chocolate Drizzle

Day 70

Breakfast: Flaxseed and Blueberry Smoothie Bowl

Lunch: Quinoa and Grilled Vegetable Buddha Bowl with Tahini Dressing

Dinner: Baked Turkey Meatloaf with Mashed Cauliflower

Snack/Dessert: Tahini and Honey Roasted Almonds

Day 71

Breakfast: Almond Butter and Banana Rice Cakes

Lunch: Sweet Potato and Black Bean Tacos with Avocado Salsa

Dinner: Roasted Brussels Sprouts with Almond-Crusted Salmon

Snack/Dessert: Peanut Butter and Coconut Balls

Day 72

Breakfast: Herb Omelet with Avocado and Arugula

Lunch: Chickpea and Spinach Stew with Coconut Milk

Dinner: Grilled Lamb Chops with Minted Quinoa Salad

Snack/Dessert: Baked Sweet Potato Chips with Paprika

Day 73

Breakfast: Pumpkin and Ginger Smoothie

Lunch: Tuna Salad with Avocado and Cucumber on Mixed Greens

Dinner: Quinoa Risotto with Mushrooms and Spinach

Snack/Dessert: Matcha and Coconut Chia Pudding

Day 74

Breakfast: Zucchini and Carrot Breakfast Fritters

Lunch: Tuna Salad with Avocado and Cucumber on Mixed Greens

Dinner: Quinoa and Roasted Vegetable Casserole with Almonds

Snack/Dessert: Pumpkin Seed and Dark Chocolate Bark

Day 30

Breakfast: Flaxseed and Blueberry Smoothie Bowl

Lunch: Chickpea and Cucumber Salad with Lemon-Tahini Dressing

Dinner: Grass-Fed Beef Stir-Fry with Ginger and Snap Peas

Snack/Dessert: Apple and Almond Butter Sandwiches

Day 31

Breakfast: Almond Butter and Banana Rice Cakes

Lunch: Baked Cod with Herb-Infused Quinoa and Asparagus

Dinner: Spaghetti Squash with Tomato Basil Sauce and Turkey Meatballs

Snack/Dessert: Ginger-Spiced Carrot Muffins

Day 32

Breakfast: Herb Omelet with Avocado and Arugula

Lunch: Red Lentil and Sweet Potato Curry with Spinach

Dinner: Vegan Chili with Sweet Potatoes and Avocado

Snack/Dessert: Mixed Berry and Chia Seed Parfait

Day 33

Breakfast: Pumpkin and Ginger Smoothie

Lunch: Grilled Chicken Salad with Mixed Berries and Walnuts

Dinner: Broiled Mackerel with Citrus Slaw and Roasted Brussels Sprouts

Lunch: Roasted Beet and Goat Cheese Salad with Walnuts

Dinner: Balsamic-Glazed Portobello Mushrooms with Zucchini Noodles

Snack/Dessert: Turmeric and Ginger Energy Balls

Day 75

Breakfast: Coconut Flour Waffles with Mixed Berries

Lunch: Grilled Salmon with Turmeric-Spiced Lentils

Dinner: Lentil and Vegetable Shepherd's Pie

Snack/Dessert: Baked Apple Slices with Cinnamon and Walnuts

Day 76

Breakfast: Matcha Smoothie with Spinach and Coconut Milk

Lunch: Quinoa and Grilled Vegetable Buddha Bowl with Tahini Dressing

Dinner: Coconut-Braised Tempeh with Bok Choy and Carrots

Snack/Dessert: Dark Chocolate-Dipped Strawberries with Pistachios

Day 77

Breakfast: Poached Eggs with Avocado and Sautéed Greens

Lunch: Grilled Shrimp Salad with Arugula and Citrus Vinaigrette

Dinner: Grass-Fed Beef Stir-Fry with Ginger and Snap Peas

Snack/Dessert: Almond Butter Stuffed Dates with Hemp Seeds

Day 78

Breakfast: Cinnamon Quinoa with Almond Milk and Cherries

Lunch: Chickpea and Cucumber Salad with Lemon-Tahini Dressing

Dinner: Grilled Eggplant with Walnut Pesto and Arugula Salad

Snack/Dessert: Coconut Macaroons with Dark Chocolate Drizzle

Day 34

Breakfast: Zucchini and Carrot Breakfast Fritters

Lunch: Roasted Carrot and Parsnip Soup with Ginger

Dinner: Seared Tuna Steak with Avocado Salad and Lime Dressing

Snack/Dessert: Tahini and Honey Roasted Almonds

Day 35

Breakfast: Coconut Flour Waffles with Mixed Berries

Lunch: Spinach and Mushroom Frittata with Sweet Potatoes

Dinner: Mediterranean Stuffed Eggplant with Feta and Pine Nuts

Snack/Dessert: Peanut Butter and Coconut Balls

Day 36

Breakfast: Matcha Smoothie with Spinach and Coconut Milk

Lunch: Black Bean and Quinoa Stuffed Zucchini Boats

Dinner: Baked Turkey Meatloaf with Mashed Cauliflower

Snack/Dessert: Baked Sweet Potato Chips with Paprika

Day 37

Breakfast: Poached Eggs with Avocado and Sautéed Greens

Lunch: Quinoa Salad with Avocado, Kale, and Pomegranate

Dinner: Roasted Brussels Sprouts with Almond-Crusted Salmon

Snack/Dessert: Matcha and Coconut Chia Pudding

Day 38

Snack/Dessert: Coconut Yogurt with Fresh Mango and Chia Seeds

Day 79

Breakfast: Almond Flour Muffins with Turmeric and Ginger

Lunch: Quinoa Salad with Avocado, Kale, and Pomegranate

Dinner: Baked Salmon with Garlic and Rosemary Sweet Potatoes

Snack/Dessert: Flaxseed Crackers with Hummus

Day 80

Breakfast: Anti-Inflammatory Smoothie with Mango, Turmeric, and Spinach

Lunch: Red Lentil and Sweet Potato Curry with Spinach

Dinner: Spaghetti Squash with Tomato Basil Sauce and Turkey Meatballs

Snack/Dessert: Oat and Date Cookies with Cinnamon

Day 81

Breakfast: Turmeric Oatmeal with Blueberries and Almonds

Lunch: Grilled Turkey Burgers with Avocado and Spinach

Dinner: Vegan Chili with Sweet Potatoes and Avocado

Snack/Dessert: Roasted Chickpeas with Paprika and Turmeric

Day 82

Breakfast: Chia Seed Pudding with Mixed Berries

Lunch: Tuna Salad with Avocado and Cucumber on Mixed Greens

Dinner: Quinoa and Roasted Vegetable Casserole with Almonds

Snack/Dessert: Turmeric-Spiced Cashew Nuts

Day 83

Breakfast: Cinnamon Quinoa with Almond Milk and Cherries

Lunch: Grilled Shrimp Salad with Arugula and Citrus Vinaigrette

Dinner: Grilled Lamb Chops with Minted Quinoa Salad

Snack/Dessert: Turmeric and Ginger Energy Balls

Day 39

Breakfast: Almond Flour Muffins with Turmeric and Ginger

Lunch: Sweet Potato and Black Bean Tacos with Avocado Salsa

Dinner: Quinoa Risotto with Mushrooms and Spinach

Snack/Dessert: Baked Apple Slices with Cinnamon and Walnuts

Day 40

Breakfast: Anti-Inflammatory Smoothie with Mango, Turmeric, and Spinach

Lunch: Chickpea and Spinach Stew with Coconut Milk

Dinner: Coconut-Braised Tempeh with Bok Choy and Carrots

Snack/Dessert: Dark Chocolate-Dipped Strawberries with Pistachios

Day 41

Breakfast: Turmeric Oatmeal with Blueberries and Almonds

Lunch: Grilled Turkey Burgers with Avocado and Spinach

Dinner: Baked Salmon with Garlic and Rosemary Sweet Potatoes

Snack/Dessert: Almond Butter Stuffed Dates with Hemp Seeds

Day 42

Breakfast: Avocado Toast with Smoked Salmon and Microgreens

Lunch: Grilled Chicken Salad with Mixed Berries and Walnuts

Dinner: Wild-Caught Cod with Sautéed Spinach and Cherry Tomatoes

Snack/Dessert: Pumpkin Seed and Dark Chocolate Bark

Day 84

Breakfast: Quinoa Breakfast Bowl with Walnuts and Pomegranate Seeds

Lunch: Roasted Carrot and Parsnip Soup with Ginger

Dinner: Seared Tuna Steak with Avocado Salad and Lime Dressing

Snack/Dessert: Apple and Almond Butter Sandwiches

Day 85

Breakfast: Greek Yogurt with Flaxseeds and Honey

Lunch: Sweet Potato and Black Bean Tacos with Avocado Salsa

Dinner: Baked Turkey Meatloaf with Mashed Cauliflower

Snack/Dessert: Ginger-Spiced Carrot Muffins

Day 86

Breakfast: Buckwheat Pancakes with Fresh Raspberries

Lunch: Grilled Shrimp Salad with Arugula and Citrus Vinaigrette

Dinner: Roasted Brussels Sprouts with Almond-Crusted Salmon

Snack/Dessert: Mixed Berry and Chia Seed Parfait

Day 87

Breakfast: Chia Seed Pudding with Mixed Berries

Lunch: Quinoa and Grilled Vegetable Buddha Bowl with Tahini Dressing

Dinner: Lentil and Vegetable Shepherd's Pie

Snack/Dessert: Coconut Yogurt with Fresh Mango and Chia Seeds

Day 43

Breakfast: Avocado Toast with Smoked Salmon and Microgreens

Lunch: Red Lentil and Sweet Potato Curry with Spinach

Dinner: Turmeric and Ginger Chicken Stir-Fry with Broccoli

Snack/Dessert: Flaxseed Crackers with Hummus

Day 44

Breakfast: Quinoa Breakfast Bowl with Walnuts and Pomegranate Seeds

Lunch: Roasted Beet and Goat Cheese Salad with Walnuts

Dinner: Wild-Caught Cod with Sautéed Spinach and Cherry Tomatoes

Snack/Dessert: Oat and Date Cookies with Cinnamon

Day 45

Breakfast: Greek Yogurt with Flaxseeds and Honey

Lunch: Chickpea and Cucumber Salad with Lemon-Tahini Dressing

Dinner: Balsamic-Glazed Portobello Mushrooms with Zucchini Noodles

Snack/Dessert: Roasted Chickpeas with Paprika and Turmeric

Breakfast: Anti-Inflammatory Green Smoothie with Kale and Pineapple

Lunch: Chickpea and Spinach Stew with Coconut Milk

Dinner: Quinoa Risotto with Mushrooms and Spinach

Snack/Dessert: Coconut Macaroons with Dark Chocolate Drizzle

Day 88

Breakfast: Cinnamon-Spiced Apple and Almond Porridge

Lunch: Quinoa and Grilled Vegetable Buddha Bowl with Tahini Dressing

Dinner: Balsamic-Glazed Portobello Mushrooms with Zucchini Noodles

Snack/Dessert: Tahini and Honey Roasted Almonds

Day 89

Breakfast: Coconut Yogurt Parfait with Chia and Hemp Seeds

Lunch: Grilled Turkey Burgers with Avocado and Spinach

Dinner: Coconut-Braised Tempeh with Bok Choy and Carrots

Snack/Dessert: Peanut Butter and Coconut Balls

Day 90

Breakfast: Flaxseed and Blueberry Smoothie Bowl

Lunch: Tuna Salad with Avocado and Cucumber on Mixed Greens

Dinner: Mediterranean Stuffed Eggplant with Feta and Pine Nuts

Snack/Dessert: Baked Sweet Potato Chips with Paprika

Congratulations On Completing The 90-Day Anti-Inflammatory Meal Plan!

Conclusion

Embarking on an anti-inflammatory diet is a powerful step toward promoting long-term health and well-being, especially for women over 60. As the body changes with age, prioritizing nutrient-dense, anti-inflammatory foods can significantly improve vitality, energy levels, and overall quality of life. By focusing on whole, unprocessed ingredients and incorporating the recipes, tips, and meal plans provided in this book, you're not only taking control of your diet but also making an investment in your future health. From the breakfasts that fuel your day, to the lunches and dinners that provide balance and nourishment, and the snacks and desserts that offer guilt-free indulgence, this journey is designed to be enjoyable, sustainable, and effective. The key is variety, consistency, and a willingness to try new things. Over time, you'll likely notice positive changes in your energy levels, digestion, joint mobility, and mental clarity, all while enjoying delicious, flavorful meals.

It's important to remember that an anti-inflammatory lifestyle isn't about perfection, but rather about making informed choices that support your body's natural healing processes. There's no one-size-fits-all approach to health, but by embracing these principles, you can create a personalized routine that fits seamlessly into your life. And remember, consistency is more impactful than occasional efforts—every step you take toward reducing inflammation will contribute to your overall well-being.

As you continue your journey, don't hesitate to revisit the meal plans, try new recipes, or modify meals to suit your preferences and needs. The goal is to create habits that last and make you feel your best every day.

Thank you for taking this step toward a healthier, more vibrant you. May the insights and recipes in this book inspire you to nourish both your body and spirit as you age with strength, grace, and vitality.

BONUS

BONUS ANTI-INFLAMMATORY DIET FOR BEGINNERS

Dear Reader,

We're thrilled to offer you our bonus "ANTI-INFLAMMATORY DIET FOR BEGINNERS"!

Simply send an email to **oliviastokes162@gmail.com**

with the subject line **BONUS ANTI-INFLAMMATORY**, and you'll receive an exclusive PDF copy of the unpublished book ANTI-INFLAMMATORY DIET FOR BEGINNERS.

This bonus guide includes <u>additional anti-inflammatory recipes</u> and a <u>30-day meal plan</u> specifically designed for beginners. It's a unique resource that will provide you with even more support and insight into your diet, giving you everything you need to continue your journey toward better health and well-being.

Dear Reader,

Thank you for choosing to explore ANTI-INFLAMMATORY DIET FOR WOMEN OVER 60. As the author, my goal is to empower women to take control of their health through nourishing, anti-inflammatory meals and balanced nutrition.

Your feedback is incredibly valuable—not only to me but also to others who are considering this book. By sharing your thoughts and experiences, you help me improve as an author and guide fellow readers on their own wellness journeys.

I would be grateful if you could take a moment to leave a review on Amazon. Whether you found the recipes helpful, the advice insightful, or have suggestions for improvement, your feedback is essential. Your insights can offer valuable direction to others looking to benefit from the anti-inflammatory lifestyle outlined in this book.

Leaving a review is simple. Just scan the QR code below with your smartphone, and you'll be taken directly to the Amazon review page. Your honest review will have a meaningful impact, and I deeply appreciate your support in helping to spread the message of health and vitality.

Thank you for being part of this journey toward a healthier, inflammation-free life.

Warm regards,

Olivia Stokes